WHAT THE HELL IS BEHAVIORAL HEALTH?

The Shell Game: A Metaphor for What is Happening to the Counseling Profession.

by

Don Hidalgo

DORRANCE
PUBLISHING CO
EST. 1920
PITTSBURGH, PENNSYLVANIA 15238

Dorrance Publishing Co
585 Alpha Drive
Pittsburgh, PA 15238
Visit our website at www.dorrancebookstore.com

ISBN: 978-1-4809-8879-8
eISBN: 978-1-4809-8833-0

This book is dedicated to my wife,

Betty Breen Hidalgo,

whose dedication and commitment to our family and our marriage in the face of my struggles with alcoholism gave birth to this book.

Acknowledgments

Louis Cataldie (Pioneer in addiction and early founder of ASAM)

David Gastfriend (First medical director of my UR services)

Gene(Deceased) and Nance Gwaltney (Corporate/personal endorsement of the value of EAP)

Tom Hagen (Deceased) (Taught me the real meaning of honesty)

Richard Heilman (Deceased) (Psychiatrist, addictionologist, mentor)

Michael Hoyt (My friend, colleague, challenger)

Paul Huffnagel (Social worker that truly understands the value of EAP's and certification)

Vernon Johnson (Deceased) (My meeting with him changed my life and career)

Doug Manship (Deceased) (More than a client he was my true friend, we shared many interests together)

Gary McGarity (Colleague who tries to keep me out of trouble in issues concerning pharmacology)

Francis Melancon (Deceased) (Union leader, Steel Workers Union, promoted our EAP as a real value to the union membership)

Paul Roman (Historian for EAP)

Kathryn Sullivan (My friend and former president of BC/BS of Louisiana, gave credibility to our EAP and UR)

Ed Silvey (Best endorser with the use of sarcasm about our EAP services)

Edwin Timmons (Deceased) (My friend and early academic endorser of EAP's)

Jon Weinberg (Deceased) (My teacher and authority on diagnostics)

Robert Whitaker (His book "Anatomy of an Epidemic" was the wake-up call for my book)

CHAPTERS

PROLOGUE

If you are one of the 600,000 mental health/substance abuse counselors/ therapists in the United States, this book is a must read. It describes in detail what is happening to your practice and income, now and in the future. The term "behavioral health" should be a major cause of concern for every person working in the mental health/substance abuse field and particularly those providing Employee Assistance Program (EAP) services. The term "behavioral health" has become universally used but the danger is that it has no real definition. This book attempts to document how the term "behavioral health" has changed the entire dynamics of the delivery of mental health services to the public in general and the EAP field in particular; and not always in the best interest of either. Thus the title "What the Hell is Behavioral Health?"

This is the story of the impact of an illness that affects every person in the United States either directly or indirectly. It is told through the eyes and experience of the founder of Hidalgo Health Associates, the oldest currently active Employee Assistance Program in the United States. The EAP is a perfect mirror of the public attitude toward alcoholism and mental health. We can see these attitudes expressed in governmental (federal and state) legislation, health insurance benefits, pharmaceuticals, and the economic cost to business.

I am grateful to all of the people cited at the front of the book. Their insight into perceptions and attitudes and their help in collecting the historical data are the foundation of my current observations and future predictions for the mental health and substance abuse fields.

CHAPTER 1

THE TELEPHONE CALL

It is the week before Thanksgiving in 1979, approximately 1:30 p.m. when my telephone rings and my secretary, Leslie, says "There is a man on the phone that insists he has to talk to you." She says, "I know you said you did not want to be disturbed but he is so insistent, as a matter of fact really hostile in his tone, that I think you had better talk to him." So I told Leslie to pass him through and let's see what's going on.

When I get on the phone he doesn't bother to introduce himself, he simply starts his conversation with "I want to hire you to come to my company and do an intervention on one of my senior managers." My response is "I don't know who you are." He says "It doesn't make any difference who I am. If you are worried about whether or not I can pay you, I can pay you." I said, "No, that's not the issue for me. I don't jump on airplanes and go do interventions unless I know it's appropriate. And at this stage of the game I know nothing about who you are or if I can even help you."

His comment then was, "I have checked around the country and have found everywhere I go, they all tell me the same thing. The person that you want to talk to is in Baton Rouge, Louisiana. His name is Don Hidalgo. That's why I am calling you."

I asked "What is your company?" He replied "Russell Corporation." Now, I knew from my personal experience with employee assistance services that Russell Corporation was a Fortune 500 company and it had an internal

1

EAP service. So my comment to him was "I know that you have an employee assistance program, why don't you use your own people to do this?" His response was "This individual is so high in the organization that I don't trust anyone to do it, I need somebody on the outside."

I commented again that I still did not have enough information to determine whether it was appropriate for me to attempt an intervention. I told him that I needed to have certain information before I could jump on a company plane and fly over to Alexander City, Alabama to do an intervention on a person that I know absolutely nothing about.

There was a pause and then the tone of his voice changed. He went from being frustrated, irritated and demanding to almost pleading when he said "If you don't come, she will die."

The person high up in the Russell organization he wanted me to do an intervention for was his wife, Nancy Russell Gwaltney. Nancy's family had founded the Russell Corporation and she was one of the principal stock holders. After hearing the desperation in Gene's voice, the following Wednesday, I found myself on the company plane flying from Baton Rouge to Alexander City, Alabama.

As an aside Nancy and her children have given me consent to use their story in the writing of this book.

The company plane arrived at the Alexander City airport just before dark. I was driven to Gene Gwaltney's office at the corporate headquarters. Gene was the president and CEO of Russell Corporation. We briefly reviewed the routine for the intervention training session scheduled for that evening and the intervention itself the following morning.

During the course of the conversation, Gene said that he did not want Nancy's parents, Mr. and Mrs. Russell, to be present because he felt Mrs. Russell would dominate the intervention.

I explained that we needed everyone who had data on Nancy's drinking, and were concerned about her well-being, to help convince her that going into treatment was the right thing to do. He was insistent that they not be present.

At this point I emphasized that everyone, including Nancy's parents, should be included in the training and actual intervention. I told Gene, "If he did not want to follow my instructions, I would not do the intervention. If he did not allow me to do the intervention on my experience that gave the best results for success, he could take me back to the airport and fly me home." As it turned out, his concerns about Mrs. Russell's attempt to control the intervention were accurate.

We met at the Russell corporate offices that evening for about 3 hours to do the intervention training. The following morning we met for the intervention at Gene and Nancy's home together with their three children, Nancy, George, and Gene, Jr. and Nancy's parents, Mr. and Mrs. Russell.

During the intervention an argument broke out between Gene and Nancy. It was at that point I realized, if I ever thought I had control of this intervention that thought was just an illusion. I leaned back, and considered what I could do to get control of this thing again and said the Lord's Prayer. About midway through the argument Nancy got up and announced that she was going to start fixing the turkey for Thanksgiving dinner. We asked her to come back. Reluctantly she came back and joined us. In the end the intervention was a success. That afternoon we were back on the airplane flying to Baton Rouge where she was admitted to the Baton Rouge General Hospital Chemical Dependency Unit (CDU).

The CDU had a policy that required that family members attend a full family week. Family week was Monday through Friday. It was a therapeutic counseling program designed to help family members understand the dynamics of an alcoholic family. It also helped them understand the recovery process, their role in the recovery process and how important their role was. So Gene and the three children came to Baton Rouge for the full week. At the end of the graduation on Friday, Gene asked to meet me for lunch before flying back to Alexander City.

At that time he was so excited about what had happened, and hopeful about the future that he asked me to put together an employee assistance program presentation for his company. I explained to him that I could not ethically do that for at least six months following a client/patient relationship either with him or with Nancy. Again in typical Gene Gwaltney fashion he said "God dammit I told you I wanted to do it now, I don't want to have to wait six months". I said "ethically that what I have to do". He replied "six months from now, write down that date, the plane is going to be at the airport picking you up to bring you back to Alexander City because I want to start this thing".

During family week the Gwaltney family had the good fortune to meet Betty Breen. Betty had been a substance abuse counselor for 17 years. At that time she had dual responsibilities both as a counselor and as the director of the family counseling services at CDU.

Betty was my wife. And as the wife of a recovering alcoholic she was intimately familiar with the issues facing the family members. She also had the remarkable ability to help the family members understand the challenges facing the patient who was in recovery. I truly believe that one of the reasons why Gene was so impressed with the program was a result of the services Betty was able to provide for them during family week.

In the history of EAP's, the story of Gene's phone call and Nancy's intervention and successful recovery is important because it provided the basis of the EAP services we initially created for the Russell Corporation which has evolved over the past forty years.

Another reason for citing this example is because both Gene and Nancy were well known in both their local community and within the textile industry. Through Gene's efforts, and Nancy's recovery, they had a positive effect on thousands of lives. There was no stigma as far as Nancy and Gene were concerned. To them alcoholism was simply an illness and it needed to be addressed. They did not hesitate to acknowledge, when appropriate that Nancy was an alcoholic and was in recovery.

I will talk later about what happened in Alexander City when we installed the EAP and what Nancy's influence was with the alcoholic community.

CHAPTER 2

MY LIFE EXPERIENCES: CHANGE BEGINS AT HOME

As I flew with Nancy back to Baton Rouge I looked down at the kaleidoscope below us, the patchwork of different geographical lines and colors that outlined the farms, the communities, the highways, and the woodlands. In some ways that image represented the same thoughts that were racing through my mind. I was thinking about the patchwork of circumstances that had profoundly changed my life since 1975.

How did I become known as an expert in this field? Why would anyone be willing to hire me to help get someone into treatment? Five years prior to 1975 I knew absolutely nothing about alcoholism. Nothing that is, other than what my wife Betty, repeatedly told me, and that was "I had a serious drinking problem." At that time I certainly did not have any professional qualifications or education other than "on the job training." It was simply my reputation as a recovering alcoholic that qualified me as a provider of intervention services.

As this book unfolds it will explore the patchwork of relationships between EAP services, the mental health industry, the physical medicine industry, the insurance industry, the pharmaceutical industry, and government regulatory agencies and legislation, both state and federal.

This is not primarily an autobiographical story but it is important that I bring you up to date on how all of this began. In order to do that I will have to give you some background on my education and work life experiences.

My college education was at Louisiana State University. The only course I had that in any way related to my future career in substance abuse was a preliminary course in Psychology. Other than that, I had no background at all in addiction and recovery. Even law school did not prepare me for what my life would be like after 1975.

When I left school I went into the life insurance business. I worked as an insurance broker specializing in estate planning and in the establishment of trusts. I was very successful in my chosen career. As a matter of fact, this success was part of my downfall. I was making a substantial amount of money and that allowed me to continue my drinking at an advanced rate.

In addition to being an active insurance agent, I also taught at LSU at the Institute of Insurance Marketing for a period of 17 years. My subject was Estate Planning and Business Insurance. I cite this because ultimately it is critical in the development of some of the EAP programs we put together. My background was further enhanced while working with the Life Underwriters Training Council (LUTC). I served on their Board of Directors and as one of their consultants providing continuity to the training and testing programs. The LUTC provided a five course program. It was the largest of its kind in the United States, with an enrollment of a quarter million students.

Additionally, I had become very active in the Life Underwriters Association and became Chairman of the Legislative Committee with the responsibility of lobbying for legislation. In 1955 there were only two requirements necessary to become a licensed life insurance agent; you had to have more than $2.00 in your pocket and you had to be able to make your mark. When I introduced my first legislation as a lobbyist I assumed all that was needed to have a bill successfully passed was "patriotism, motherhood, and apple pie." I was quickly introduced to the world of vested interests.

It immediately became obvious that the smaller life insurance companies were strongly against this new legislation. The president of one of these companies testified "if you pass this bill you will put us out of business because many of our people are just school bus drivers and they are not educated to the point where they can read all these whereas and wherefores." On that point I decided that I would not testify and let the committee make its own decision concerning the requirements to be a qualified agent.

This bill was actually passed and we now have legislation that requires a written examination for life insurance, property and casualty agents. Ultimately my legislative and lobbying activities would be expanded when I became active in the addiction field.

When I returned home from treatment in 1976 I began to receive phone calls from people saying "you don't know me but, we would like for you to talk to our father, mother, brother, janitor, or president. They have a serious alcohol problem and we understand that you are able to help convince them to go to treatment." The help I provided was called *intervention*. Hidalgo Health Associates was initially established on providing intervention services.

As a result of those calls, I began to do interventions and subsequently needed a place that I could refer people for treatment. The Baton Rouge General Hospital had opened a chemical dependency unit in 1976. I went to them and asked if they would accept my patients and we became one of the major sources of their patient body. I had no financial interest in CDU. I sent them patients because they gave us a good program and good results.

After about a year, it became obvious that my time was being consumed with the volunteer work of doing interventions and talking to the business community about the problem of alcohol and drugs in the workplace. I decided at that point that I wanted to be more than an administrator and in order to do that I had to have more education in this field of addiction and recovery.

At that time we did not have any educational programs in the state of Louisiana that addressed the issues of substance abuse. Unfortunately, even today, we have a very limited number of programs at our major universities that deal with addiction training for counselors, psychologists, social workers, LPC's and marriage and family therapists.

The University of Minnesota at that time was, and still is, one of the major universities that provided specific training in the field of addiction. I applied for and was accepted to the Department of Counseling in a limited program focused on addiction and was fortunate to study under Dr. Jon Weinberg. Dr. Weinberg was a tall, gaunt Scandinavian who had all the personality of a dead fish. Yet, he was an absolute genius when it came to diagnostics. Still to this day, I have all of his monographs on how to conduct a successful interview for diagnostic purposes.

One key comment that Dr. Weinberg made over and over again that has stuck in my mind through the years was, "It is not how the patient answers your question, it's how they reframe the question to move it into the area where they can anticipate what you are looking for or put them in a more favorable light."

For example; I would ask, "Do you drink daily"? Or if I would ask "How much do you drink" the patient would reframe the question by asking "What do you mean when you say, how much do you drink?" "What do you mean when you say "drink daily"?

I remember one particular attorney I was working with. After about three hours of asking him questions and he reframing my questions, I turned to him and said "Counselor if you were a juror and I was the attorney trying to present the case you had given me how would you vote on this?" He smiled and said "I don't guess I would come out too favorable on that". I said "then why don't we cut to the chase so we can get to the point, get you help with this problem"? To this day every time I do an evaluation on a patient I hear Dr. Weinberg talking in my head "listen to how the question is reframed".

Another influential person I met was Dr. Richard Heilman, M.D. He was the consulting psychiatrist for the Hazelden Foundation where I went to treatment for my own alcohol problem. I recall the first time I heard Dr. Heilman give a talk. He arrived late for the session. It had been snowing and his comment was "that he knew this was going to be a bad day because he overslept that morning. He then went outside and found his car had a flat tire. He then decided he would call the suicide line to tell them why he was running late and see what was going on. When he called, the message on the answering machine was "go to hell".

I was immediately attracted to Dr. Heilman when I heard him speak. In the course of that first one hour talk, he opened the door to the realization that I was dealing with something beyond my will power and that alcoholism was in fact an illness. For a number of years I had agonized over why it was that I could not control the amount I was drinking since I was by nature, self-disciplined. His first talk was the beginning of my recovery and my introduction to the field of addiction.

Subsequent to when I was discharged from Hazelden, I called Dr. Heilman and asked if he would allow me to serve as an intern with him at the VA hospital in Minneapolis-St. Paul. He accepted my application and I did complete an internship with him.

I can still remember when we were making rounds, he would turn to all of us and in his own style would say "Now if any of you hotshots think you're good enough to handle an alcoholic/addict by yourself, you better have a damn good psychiatrist of your own, because they will drive you crazy." That comment confirmed that one- on- one counseling does not help for an alcoholic.

Dr. Heilman's studies on mice and the effect of dopamine or lack of dopamine in the brain were the basis of my becoming deeply involved in the chemical and medical aspects of this illness.

I am eternally grateful to both Dr. Heilman and Dr. Weinberg for the help that they gave me. Much of my career has hinged on their work. I attempted to reach out to them and share some of the information I was going to incorporate in the book. Unfortunately both had already passed away.

CHAPTER 3

INTERVENTION: MINE AND OTHERS'

Like many of us that chose to go into this field I am a recovering alcoholic. My wife and I had seven children together so I wasn't drunk all the time. At least I did seven good things.

My educational and business background did not lead to my becoming involved in the employee assistance services. Yet my life experiences all lead up to December 14, 1975, the day my family did an intervention which resulted in my going to treatment at Hazelden in Minnesota.

My alcoholism had gotten completely out of hand when Betty, my wife, said to me one morning at breakfast "Right now we have two crazy parents in this house and we need to have at least one sane one to raise these three children who are still at home. Don, you are going to have to agree to get help or leave because we can't keep going like this." I accepted her statement as an ultimatum and decided that the best course of action was to move out. By leaving I thought that I would teach her a lesson; that she really needed me and my problem was not nearly as severe as she thought it was.

One afternoon I had just returned from lunch when my secretary Leslie came in with the telephone messages. This was in the old days when telephone messages were still delivered by voice and messages were subsequently written by hand. In other words it was pre-voice mail, pre- email. As Leslie handed me the messages she said "I think this is one that you need to answer first, it's from Betty."

We did not normally talk to each other during our separation except on occasion when there was something to do with the children or our finances. When I called Betty, she asked me to meet her on Thursday evening at 7:00 at the Catholic Life Center. She said we had some things to discuss and that would be the most convenient location. Little did I realize the profound effect and the profound change which would occur in my life as a result of the meeting that Thursday night.

The speaker that Betty wanted to hear was Dr. Vernon Johnson. Dr. Johnson, in my opinion, created the concept of the modern intervention process as described in his book *"I'll Quit Tomorrow"*.

This book walks the reader through the disease of alcoholism presenting its symptoms and behavior in layman's terms. It also describes the dynamics of the relationships between the alcoholic, their spouse, family, and friends and their reluctance to take action. In other words – it illustrates the need to educate and intervene the interveners before you get to the patient. For a deeper understanding of how interventions work I suggest you read Dr. Johnson's book.

I arrived at the Catholic Life Center early and had the opportunity to meet with Dr. Johnson and speak with him prior to the meeting. While at the seminar I bought his book. He autographed it for me and I still have it to this day. The autograph read "To Don, on our joint journey on the road to recovery. With best wishes and good luck, Vernon."

During my separation from Betty, the children would come to visit me at my apartment. On one occasion I sent my copy of "I'll Quit Tomorrow" home with my son Bill. I told him it was all about alcoholism and to give it to his mother. I thought since she was so bent out of shape about the subject she would find it fascinating reading. When my intervention ended, I turned to Betty and asked "Where did you come up with this goofy idea?" Her response was, "in that book you gave me." I asked "what book?" She replied the "I'll Quit Tomorrow" book. Then I began to realize when I questioned her in more detail, I had only read chapters 1 through 4 which talked about the illness. Chapters 5 through 13, which I hadn't read, talked about the intervention. I am firmly convinced that I unintentionally set up my own intervention when I gave her that book.

Suffice it to say, Betty took the advice in Dr. Johnson's book seriously. The intervention was done with all seven of my children and two of my former students, Vince Bellepani with Penn Mutual Life Insurance and Bill Smith with Lincoln National Life. They were at the time, competitors of mine in the insurance business.

My intervention did not go well. I was the typical angry, hostile, defensive alcoholic that you usually find in a pre-intervention situation. The one thing I can say, that was different about my intervention, was that my family was absolute in their decision. They were convinced that if I did not go to treatment that I would wind up either becoming brain dead as a result of the blackouts or that I would commit suicide.

During the intervention process, when they completed telling me what their concerns were, I thanked them all for coming to my office, and then told them "to get the hell out". The problem was they didn't get the hell out. I remember Michael, my oldest son, looked at me and said "Dad, whether you realize it or not, alcohol is killing you and it's taking us with you. And we're not going there anymore. If you don't go into treatment we're going to get a commitment order and have you committed to a treatment center".

At that point I said to him "Michael you do remember that I went to law school. You think you know a little about the law? I'm going to teach you something now, real quick. I'll meet you in the middle of a courtroom. We will have an interdiction hearing and then we will see who is determined to be crazy." (The interdiction is a legal process in which a court is asked to determine whether a person is intellectually capable of conducting their own affairs). I challenged Michael and said that he couldn't get a commitment on me since I did not fit the criteria of what a person would look or behave like if they were incapable of managing their affairs. I made it clear that most of the judges in Baton Rouge were friends, former classmates, or clients of mine, and the coroner, Dr. Hypolite Landry, was a personal friend.

The way I controlled my family over the years was with the checkbook. So at that point I said to them "all of you who are in college or private school, you can find another way to get your education; because as of today I'm closing the checkbook. You are out on your own. And Betty, there will be no more money for you either."

Michael looked at me and said "Dad you are going to do what you are going to do and we are going to do what we have got to do. But we cannot, we will not let this continue on." I suppose it was at that point that I realized I really didn't have too many options other than do the courtroom appearance.

And I certainly did not want to do that as it would be a source of embarrassment to me in this community.

As the intervention continued, a little voice went off in the back of my mind and said "is it that bad and you can't see it?" My biggest problem was that I was a "functional alcoholic". I was still able to successfully operate my financial and insurance business. I got up and went to work every day. So how could I have a problem that was so bad that I had to go off to a treatment center? I finally came to the conclusion that everything else I had tried didn't work so why not this. Although, I didn't believe that the treatment program they were proposing was going to be any different from anything else that I had already done to deal with my alcoholism.

So what is an intervention? There are many different definitions but the one that I use is; an intervention is an appropriate process in which other people intervene in a person's life to help them when their health or life is threatened.

What is the purpose of the intervention? Due to the progressive and debilitating nature of addiction, the person is often not even aware that their behavior is out of control. So the purpose of the intervention is twofold; to express the concern others have for the person and to make absolutely clear to the alcoholic/addict the destructive nature of their behavior and the disastrous affect it is having on their life and the life of those around them.

Most of the time we think of interventions as being strictly for alcohol and drug addiction. However, I have done interventions for other issues that were equally life and health threatening. One such case was a person who was morbidly obese. If you had listened to the scripts you would have thought that the people were talking about alcoholism. I have also done interventions on people who are diabetic and were not taking their insulin. Their reasoning for not wanting to change was that, "if they had to continue to stick that needle in their stomach every day they would just as soon be dead." I have also done interventions on people with gambling addictions.

Before the intervention, the people involved often need assistance to break through the commonly held myths surrounding addiction. One such seemingly irrefutable myth is "you can't help someone who refuses to be helped" or stated another way "you can lead a horse to water but you can't make em' drink." However, there is a part that's left out and that is "you can't make em' drink, but you can let them smell the water and make em' thirsty". Another common myth is that an intervention is an ambush. More to the point, the intervention is not an attack on the patient, it is not a "gotcha" program, it is not a lynch mob, or a hanging crew. If it comes across in that fashion it will not be effective.

The intervention is designed primarily to break through the denial system that protects the alcoholic/addict from seeing their real behavior. A successful intervention is based on the care and concern of those doing the intervention. And the key to an intervention is not when you meet with the patient but rather the pre-intervention process of educating and preparing the people doing the intervention. So in effect, you have to intervene on the interveners before you even get to the patient.

Many of our interventions are conducted as a result of work situations on behalf of our EAP clients. In preparation for the intervention I first meet with the family, friends, and employers. We talk about what their concerns are and I try to get a picture of the severity of the problem. I explain to them that the success of an intervention depends on how well they communicate their care and concerns to the patient. I teach them how to write very specific scripts describing the alcoholic/addicts behavior, how it makes them feel and the affects that behavior has on their lives. It is essential that they understand how to present this material in a factual and non-judgmental way.

So in effect, the focus is on how the behavior of the alcoholic/addict affects the people who are doing the intervention rather than the alcoholic/addict themselves.

The pre-intervention meetings are normally held on Monday or Tuesday afternoon with the intervention scheduled for the next day. Most of the interventions are done first thing in the morning in the home of the person we are intervening. The presumption is that the person is going into treatment and by doing them in the morning we have enough time to transport the patient to a treatment center. Before the intervention a reservation is made at a treatment center that has been chosen for this particular patient's needs. This is done in consort with the family and the employer based on insurance and other factors.

The intervention itself is divided into three stages: The first stage is when a patient walks in and sees who is there. Most of the time they are aware of what's going to happen, they just don't understand how it is going to happen. I explain to them that first we are going to present the group's concerns. The second stage is when we ask them to sit and listen to the scripts that are going to be read. I let them know they don't have to agree with what they hear, but ask instead, that they simply just listen and process the information. The last stage is when everyone has read their scripts and I turn to the patient and say "you have heard about their concerns and what the problems are. We come to you this morning with a solution to the problem. We have made arrangements for you to go into a treatment center, will you go with us today?" The statement is always with an emphasis on "today".

Rarely does a patient ever respond at that point and say "ok I'll go." Most of the time this is when the real intervention begins. We take every objection put forward by the patient as valid, regardless of how unrealistic it maybe. We attempt to convince the person to take advantage of the treatment offered. Here are a few of the more common objections by the patient, "I don't have a problem". "I can't take time off to go to treatment". "I will go see a psychiatrist". "I don't think all the concerns of my family are valid." When an employer is doing the intervention you might hear, "Are you going to fire me if I don't go to treatment" or "Who's going to know I am in treatment for alcoholism."

There are three ways that people go to treatment. The first one is voluntarily. This is rare but does occur when a person has this sudden insight into what their behavior is and how severe it has become. They voluntarily pick up the phone and check themselves into a treatment center. The second way people go into treatment is the result of an intervention by the family, friends, and employer. They go because they have been coerced or loved into getting help (which was what helped me). The third way is when all other efforts have failed and there is a valid concern about the safety of self and others. A commitment order can be executed that requires a person to be placed in a treatment center. The commitment order must demonstrate that the person is a danger to themselves or others. Some jurisdictions define this in a strict interpretation and others on a much broader basis.

The question is "which of these three ways ultimately turns out to be the most successful?" Your first response might be that the person going in voluntarily is the one that is going to be most successful. The exact opposite is often true.

This person has neither been confronted with their behavior nor has the denial system begun to be broken down. So when treatment begins to push the person to confront their behavior, which would normally have been done in an intervention, they decide "I don't need to be here."

The second one is where the person goes into treatment but goes as a result of the intervention but not the legal commitment. The only difference between a person who is legally committed and a person who goes in "as a result of an intervention" is about three to five days. That's about how long the anger lasts before the person finally settles down and decides that "Well, maybe while I'm here I had just soon do something about it."

I began doing interventions when I returned from treatment at Hazelden. Over the past forty years I have conducted over two thousand interventions, sometimes as many as three or four in a day.

When people approach me about doing an intervention they often ask me, "What is your success rate?" My first reaction is "What do you mean by success?" If by success you mean how many people have we done an intervention for and how many have actually gone to treatment? That is one statistic. If you are talking about how many people have gone to treatment and remained abstinent after treatment that is a separate statistic.

Let me answer the first question about the success of the intervention going into treatment. Of the roughly two thousand interventions I have personally conducted, there were fifty seven that did not get up, get in a car, or get on an airplane, and go to a treatment center as requested. The way I explain to the family and friends about the statistics and the success rate is that if your patient is one of those two thousand plus that went to treatment, then for you it is one hundred percent successful. On the other hand, if your patient is one that did not go to treatment, then for you that is one hundred percent failure. So I would rather not give you the statistics. What you need to be concentrating on is; do your best to help them and see what happens after that.

The success of an intervention is predicated on the preparation, commitment and support that the family, friends, and employer will give during the intervention.

The following cases were selected as examples of interventions to illustrate a specific need or requirement for a successful intervention.

Case #1: The Mirror Wife

One of my most unusual interventions dealt with a bi-polar wife. The husband's employer called me about his behavior. It fit the classic profile of unexplained absenteeism, deteriorating job performance, emergency phone calls, and borrowing money. On the surface it appeared the employee had the problem, however as I investigated the data prior to the intervention it became obvious the problem was with the wife and the husband was a mirror of her behavior. She was a member of the Christian Science church and had refused to take medication for her bi-polar condition. I anticipated this as a resistance and sought the help of her reader (reader means minister in other denominations) to participate in the intervention. We were successful in getting her to agree to treatment and to use medication.

Case #2: Double Barrel

I had performed about twenty-five or thirty interventions when I did this one. I was requested by a woman to do an intervention on her sister and brother-in-law, both of whom were alcoholics and were in business together. The intervention group consisted of the couple's three children (ages 20, 16, and 12) an aunt, uncle and friend. I couldn't finish the intervention. I learned that to intervene on two people at the same time, does not work. However, the husband and wife both agreed that if they ever drank again, they would go to treatment.

When this intervention was concluded and I was driving back to Baton Rouge I began thinking about the success or the failure of the interventions that I had done. Until that time every person that I had conducted an intervention on had gone to treatment. I realized that subconsciously I was taking credit for getting these people to agree to go. Now, if I was going to take credit for them going, I would have to take the responsibility for them not going. This was a wake-up call for me and made me realize that I was not the one achieving this result. It was a combination of three things: one, it was the support and the preparation of the interveners, second, it was the level of pain the person was in, and third, it was at the grace and assistance from a higher power.

There is an unusual ending to this particular intervention. Approximately a year from the date that we did the intervention I got a phone call from the husband and he said "Don I would like to go to treatment, would you get me in somewhere." I called him back and said that I had a bed for him and his wife. "She will not be coming with me," he stated. I assumed this meant she was still opposed to going to treatment. Instead he told me she had died the previous month from cirrhosis. So how do you constitute the success or the lack of success on that case? Initially I put it down as a failure.

Case #3: Hypnosis

I received a phone call from a psychiatrist asking me if I would intervene on one of his patients. This particular psychiatrist had attended one of my classes on conducting an intervention so he knew of me and what services I performed. I followed the usual format of bringing the family together and included the psychiatrist as well. At the end of the intervention the patient turned to him and he said "Doctor I thought we had agreed that I was doing better. I thought we had agreed that you would hypnotize me to where I would only have two glasses of wine in the evening." The psychiatrist looked at him and said "that was the agreement. The problem is that you are now drinking a full bottle of wine which equates to about five glasses, so the hypnosis did not work. I recommend that you follow Don's advice and go to treatment."

Case #4: The Butterfly Man

I was requested by the CEO of a major oil exploration company and the family (in this case nine children) to perform an intervention on the chairman of this man's company. I knew the morning that I drove into the family compound and saw Mercedes, BMW's, and Bentley's that this was not the usual intervention. I subsequently found out that all of the children arrived in their own Learjet's to do the intervention. When I walked into the house that morning the patient looked around and said "Whose birthday is it?" and I wanted to laugh to myself and say "It's yours and you are not even aware of it." In AA, the day that we have our last drink is considered to be our sobriety birthday. During the course of that intervention when the fifth or sixth child was reading their script for their Dad he said "Okay I give up, I'll go".

The interesting thing about this case is that subsequently he would call me about contemporaries of his with whom he had investments and ask me to conduct an intervention on them. He often referred to me as "The Butterfly Man" as though I had a butterfly net and we were going to go catch the butterflies/patients and put them in treatment. He actually had a piece of jewelry made in the form of a butterfly net for me.

Case #5: Intervention in the Middle of the North Sea

I was contracted by an international oil company to do an intervention on one of their drilling engineers. They were having serious production problems as a result of his drinking. As it turned out when they flew me out to the drilling platform a storm was approaching. As a result I had to stay aboard the rig for three days before we actually got started on the intervention. This was interesting in that there was no way for this guy to leave partly because of the storm and partly due to the fact that we had to fly in and out of there with a helicopter. This intervention was successful, he did go to treatment, and he is still in recovery as far as I know.

Case #6: The Politician's Wife

I was asked to do an intervention on a politician's wife who had a serious alcohol and prescription drug problem. This was one of the marathon cases we started early in the morning and did not finish until about four o'clock in the afternoon. This was also one of the cases where we had to use a judicial commitment. I remember looking at the lady and saying, "I don't think you understand how severe the problem is, so based on that, we have got a commitment that is going to require that you go to treatment." She looked at me and said "Do what the hell you've got to do but I'm not going anywhere". So with that, the police came, put her in handcuffs, and physically took her to treatment.

About a week after she was in treatment I just happened to be visiting the treatment center to check on one of my other patients and she walked by and spoke to me. I asked the counselor "Who is that lady?" and they responded "That is one of your patients." I was absolutely astounded. I did not recognize her. I realized that when people get into recovery they not only change psychologically but physically as well. When we did the intervention she was an old shrewish looking woman with real anger and hatred in her face that was reflected in her whole body. This was just a week after the intervention and her body had relaxed and there must have been at least ten or fifteen years that dropped off from her face. I knew then that there were many other benefits from doing an intervention.

Case #7: Commitment Laws

I got a phone call from one of my clients asking me to assist him and some of his contemporaries in helping one of their competitors. The patient happened to be a close friend of the client. This particular case involved a man who was the President/CEO of a major New York Stock Exchange company. I always try to do my homework in advance before I go out of state and this was an out of state intervention.

The morning that we did the intervention there were no family members present, only his business associates and a judge. We did the intervention with the patient still lying in bed. He was severely hung over. After we finished doing the presentation of the concerns, he announced to me "You and your offer of help can go straight to hell, I'm not going anywhere." I then mentioned something about a commitment and he sat up and said "I know the law as well as you do and you can't commit me unless you get a judge to sign a commitment order." I said "put your robe on and pull the drapes back from the other room." When he did this there was a judge sitting there. Bear in mind this group of people had all kind of influence that would not normally be available to us. The judge said "I have heard what the concerns are and I will issue a commitment." To which he replied "By the time you are able to execute that commitment I'll be on the company jet and I'll be in South America where there is no extradition agreement." At which point I suggested that he look out the window, there were two state police cruisers sitting there, and I told him, "You have a choice, you can either go to treatment or you can go to the psychiatric hospital" (which had a terrible reputation in that particular state). I cite this case to point out the fact that if you are not prepared for as many contingencies as possible you can lose the patient at the last minute.

Case #8: The Doctor's Friends

I was asked by a physician to perform an intervention on one of his friends, who also happened to be a physician and partner. There were two dentists, two other physicians, and several nurses that were involved in this intervention. No family members participated. During the course of the training period when we were talking about the groups concerns about the patient's behavior I would say "hold up the mirror so the patient can see what it is you are truly concerned about." Halfway through this process several of them in the room looked around and said almost simultaneously "you know what, I think I am describing myself, when I am talking to him." My comment to them is always the same. "This is about him, not about you. If he confronts you about the fact that you drink or behave the same way he does, you acknowledge it. You can deal with your problem after the intervention and make a decision about what you are going to do."

Subsequently one of the physicians, two of the nurses, and one of the dentists actually went into treatment and into recovery. This, however, happened as a result of attending AA meetings not through an intervention.

Case #9: The Blackout

I was contacted by a hospital administrator because of their concern about one of their physicians, a cardiologist. He had begun to develop serious problems which were being carried over into the operating room. The event that precipitated the call for an intervention was that while the doctor was performing a heart catheterization he lost the needle and didn't know what to do.

The blackout is an interesting phenomenon related to alcoholism. Alcohol directly interferes with new long and short term memory creation. As long as it is a routine procedure the alcoholic can do it without even being aware. We can be in a blackout and continue to function as though we were actually aware of what is going on. In this case, however, a different situation presented itself. He had never lost a needle before and he didn't know what to do or how to respond. It was a good thing that he had an excellent nurse standing by because she was able to retrieve the needle and save the patient.

We did a successful intervention. The patient went into treatment. However, he relapsed within ninety days and within a year he died of an overdose on medications. All of the interventions that result in treatment don't necessary lead to a successful recovery.

Case #10: Alcoholics Lie

I did an intervention at the request of Nancy Gwaltney on a physician she knew. This is an example of how active she became in the alcoholic community following her recovery. I questioned the patient about his last drink or use of medications. It's a good thing that I remembered alcoholics/addicts lie. I had originally intended to charter a plane and fly the patient to the treatment center myself. I had a pilot's license since the age of 14. At the last minute I changed my mind and chartered a flight with a pilot. Two hours later and 15,000 feet in the air my patient went into withdrawal seizures. If I had been flying the plane we would have crashed. I always carried a pint of whiskey with me for just such occasions.

Case #11: The 5 Year Old Son

This case is important to prove that young children are affected by a parent's alcoholism. The father was a big man (6'7") who was a heavy equipment operator. The wife came to me initially wanting to know when an intervention was needed. Typically the spouse does not want to admit there is a problem until something dramatic happens. She called to ask if the following incident was important enough to have an intervention. Her husband was drunk and drove a DC16 bulldozer through the company parking lot crushing 5 automobiles. I said, "Now was a good time to intervene."

During the intervention, the last person to present their concerns was their five year old son who said "papa when I hear you fuss at mama, when you are drinking that old beer, I get scared and crawl under the bed. At Thanksgiving you were drinking that old beer and you got mad and threw the turkey out into the yard. The dog ate our turkey. I don't want to be scared and hide under the bed anymore."

As an indication of how successful and how prominent the use of interventions had become was when former President Gerald Ford decided to do an intervention on his wife, Betty Ford. She had become addicted to alcohol and was abusing prescription medications. It was reported that there were four professionals on the short list to conduct the intervention, they were: Dr. Vernon Johnson, Dr. Paul Concanon, Don Hidalgo, and Lt. Comm. Pat Benedict (RN).

The selection of a woman, Lt. Commander Benedict, was the right choice for this intervention since female alcoholics tend to feel a higher degree of shame regarding their alcoholism. This is reinforced by the negative public perception that holds women being drunk in a different light than their male counterparts. Women often cite psychological or medical problems as the cause for their use.

I was one of the three people responsible for the passing of the commitment laws for substance abuse in the state of Louisiana. At the time, I worked with Dr. Hypolite Landry, the coroner of East Baton Rouge Parish and Judge Luther Cole who presided over the 19th Judicial District. On their advice, I drafted the legislation that was submitted to the judicial committee at the state legislature. Judge Cole accompanied us to the presentation and I remember remarking to him afterwards that as a lobbyist I would have appreciated an opportunity to have him present every time that I had a bill. Because of Judge Cole we were well received and the bill went through exactly as was proposed.

What did Hidalgo Health Associates help to create in the EAP field? We were the first, and perhaps today, the only major EAP that still includes interventions as part of our contract for EAP services. There are a couple of reasons for this. Very few people are trained in the intervention process and most EAP companies are not willing to spend the time, energy, and money to provide this kind of a service.

Other barriers for companies may be that they are not convinced of the effectiveness of an intervention and treatment or perhaps they fear potential legal consequences. On average it takes about six to eight hours of preliminary preparation and training and two to six hours for the actual intervention itself. This means a total of anywhere from ten to fifteen hours that have to be devoted to an intervention.

In summary, as the reader of this book, what is your attitude towards an intervention? As one employer described it; it's an ambush. Do you have a negative view of the intervention process or do you see this as a beneficial therapeutic process that enables a better outcome for the patient?

CHAPTER 4

HISTORY OF ALCOHOLISM

This story cannot be told without a brief historical review of alcohol in American society and in particular the American workplace. This book requires a review of societal and personal attitudes toward the words: *alcohol and drugs*. Drugs will be discussed in a subsequent chapter.

My description of attitude is "how people behave based on their own core values and belief system when they hear certain words". In large part it is the image of the word that is conveyed rather than the definition of the word (this is based on a study called semantics). Very few of us, and society in general, have a neutral attitude toward alcohol and drugs.

The following story illustrates best the attitude describing this problem of neutrality. As you read this story about the "Whiskey Speech", I challenge you to think about which side you fall on when you look at your own attitude towards the author's description of alcohol and the alcoholic.

The following speech was delivered by Judge Noah S. Sweat, nicknamed "Soggy". Judge Sweat was a Mississippi legislator, judge, and college professor. He gave this speech during the deliberation of whether the state of Mississippi should continue its prohibition of alcohol. It is considered to be a classic in double speak on this issue.

"My friends,
"I had not intended to discuss this controversial subject at this

particular time. However, I want you to know that I do not shun controversy. On the contrary, I will take a stand on any issue at any time, regardless of how fraught with controversy it might be. You have asked me how I feel about whiskey. All right, here is how I feel about whiskey.

"If when you say whiskey you mean the devil's brew, the poison scourge, the bloody monster, that defiles innocence, dethrones reason, destroys the home, creates misery and poverty, yea, literally takes the bread from the mouths of little children; if you mean the evil drink that topples the Christian man and woman from the pinnacle of righteous, gracious living into the bottomless pit of degradation, and despair, and shame and helplessness, and hopelessness, then certainly I am against it.

"But;

"If when you say whiskey you mean the oil of conversation, the philosophic wine, the ale that is consumed when good fellows get together, that puts a song in their hearts and laughter on their lips, and the warm glow of contentment in their eyes; if you mean Christmas cheer; if you mean the stimulating drink that puts the spring in the old gentleman's step on a frosty, crispy morning; if you mean the drink which enables a man to magnify his joy, and his happiness, and to forget, if only for a little while, life's great tragedies, and heartaches, and sorrows; if you mean that drink, the sale of which pours into our treasuries untold millions of dollars, which are used to provide tender care for our little crippled children, our blind, our deaf, our dumb, our pitiful aged and infirm; to build highways and hospitals and schools, then certainly I am for it.

"This is my stand. I will not retreat from it. I will not compromise."

"When I finished the first half of the speech, there was a tremendous applause. The second half of the speech, after the close of which, the wets all applauded. The drys were as unhappy with the second part of the speech as the wets were with the first half," he said.

The Clarion Ledger, Saturday, February 24, 1996, Jackson, MS, p. 3B.

Which group would you have identified with—the wet or dry?

The story of the EAP is best told through the history and development of civilization's attitude towards alcohol. Probably, the first civilization to discover alcohol were the Neanderthals. It is not hard to visualize the Neanderthals reaction to the discovery of a fruit that had fermented producing alcohol. Their faces would have expressed surprise, pleasure, excitement at the mind altering effect of this fruit. Thus, mankind was introduced to alcohol.

Humans seem to have an innate curiosity about altered states of the mind and began a love-hate relationship with the product that produces that condition.

There was a recent discovery of containers in Northern China going back eleven thousand years ago. These containers housed evidence of a liquid stored there containing alcohol. We know from historical fact that beer was developed some four thousand years ago by the Samarians and the Egyptians.

In order to understand how alcohol is viewed by society it's important that we have a history of the three major forms of alcohol that have been utilized over the last thousands of years. By looking at these types of alcohol we can gain a clearer prospective as to how society's attitudes have been formed towards either the positive or negative about the societal and religious use of alcohol. Over many centuries those attitudes have changed dramatically and I will elaborate later on how all this came together in the formation of the EAPs. The three types of alcohol that society and man have perfected and currently use are beer, wine, and distilled alcohol, i.e. gin and other forms of "hard liquor".

Beer
The history of beer goes back four thousand years to the Samarians and the Egyptians. The Samarians actually used beer as a form of religious worship and the priests that were in charge of brewing the beer were considered to be sacred messengers of the Gods. The Egyptians believed Tanenet was the Goddess of Beer. The area in Northern Africa referred to as the Golden Crescent was the ideal place for the beginning of beer for it had a combination of three things that were necessary in order for beer to come into existence. One, the geography and the climate had to be conducive to the production of barley and wheat. Second, you had to have a roving nomadic society that was collecting and using different forms of grain. Third, human curiosity and circumstance.

The modern day version of a barroom was exemplified by some of the paintings in the Egyptian tombs which showed people standing next to a large container about waist high that held beer. One of the problems that you have is that all of the residue from the barley, hops, and wheat would float to the surface and in order to be able to drink this beer you had to have a way to get down to the bottom of the container. This was also a problem in the 1920's and 30's making home brew. The Egyptians took hallowed out reeds, resembling long tubes, which they inserted into the container and they would stand there and drink. In effect we got the first standing bar for drinking beer. This is probably the first example of "belly-up to the bar".

Beer played a significant role in the daily diets of the people in the medieval period in the eighth, ninth, and tenth centuries. During that time, with the increase in the development of cities, pollution became a severe problem causing a lack of drinkable water. Therefore beer was usually drank in lieu of water, and was considered to be a part of the natural food process. This had a particular impact with the Black (Death) Plague which wiped out roughly twenty five percent of the population of Europe at that time. Contaminated water was one of the suspected causes of the Black Plague, however recent discoveries indicate it was probably caused by rats, infected by fleas, which were aboard sailing vessels moving from port to port.

Additionally, beer was also reported to have had hundreds of medicinal uses as well. The following is taken from an article published in "Activebeat" titled "10 Ways Drinking Beer Can Help Save Your Life." Some medicinal benefits listed were: reduce blood pressure, reduce chances of a heart attack, stimulate the brain, as an antiseptic, and to strengthen bones. In the medieval periods from the fifteenth to the seventeenth centuries beer was primarily produced in the monasteries by the Monks. Here is a famous satire set to song about how monks drank beer or wine:

> *"To drink like a Capuchin is to drink poorly; to drink like a Benedictine is to drink deeply; to drink like a Dominican is pot after pot; but to drink like a Franciscan is to drink the cellar dry."*

Earlier we talked about the original brewing of beer by accident or circumstance. The following principles of brewing applied to the original discovery. The brewing of beer can be a relatively simple affair. A grain, usually barley, is wet thus causing it to sprout, it is allowed to dry, and then is roasted. An additional washing process creates a thick sweet liquid which is then boiled. Year's later hops was added for flavoring and then subsequently other fruits and spices.

With the introduction of yeast, intentionally or accidentally, into the brewing process, a brewer once commented "when the bad little yeast boys came into the beer brew they started farting in our brewery which now created a new gas".

There are religious convictions on alcohol in general and beer in particular. Beer had a particular religious significance both in the Catholic Church and in the Protestant Reformation. Martin Luther and John Calvin were contemporaries during the Protestant Reformation, they viewed beer as an important economic resource, and this influenced their religious attitude towards beer as being something that was a "gift from God". This was different than the attitudes of the later religious abolitionists who condemned the use of alcohol.

The Pilgrims are credited with the introduction of beer into the United States. They came to the New World carrying forty thousand gallons of beer as ballast for their ships. When they got to the New England coast they knew that they would run out of beer and since it provided valuable sustenance that was needed to survive, one of the first things they did upon landing was to build a brewery.

In March 1621 at the Plymouth Colony, a group of Indians appeared from the edge of the woods and among them was a tall Indian in native garb named Samoset. He walked up to the Pilgrims and in perfect English says "Do you have beer?" The Pilgrims were astounded by this question. Samoset had been in contact with English fishermen, learned the English language from them, and was introduced to beer.

Beer was considered the poor man's drink. There is an interesting historical fact that says that one of the conditions outlined in the Magna Carta (Clause 35) was that there would be a purity of ale and wine and an adequacy of supply. Clause 35 reads:

> "Let there be throughout our kingdom a single measure for wine and a single measure for ale and a single measure for corn, namely the London quarter."

Beer became a very popular drink because it contained a much lower alcohol content and it could be drank in moderation much easier than could the higher alcohol content of gin or wine.

Wine

Historically, it was probably the Neanderthals that also discovered the first presentation of wine or some other fermented fruit. We specifically know that the Greeks referred to the use of wine as being a gift from the gods, but for anyone who abused the wine, that was considered to be in violation of Greek values. The Greeks were the first ones to develop a sophisticated system of philosophy to explain man, mathematics, and the universe and would condemn anything interfering with the brains ability to be able to reason.

Like the Greeks, the Romans were also very critical of anyone who drank to excess. As a matter of fact they refer to anyone who became drunk off of wine as a "Graper".

One of the great historical figures reported to have had a "Graper" problem was St. Monica, the mother of St. Augustine. If genetics holds true this was also one of the reasons why St. Augustine had a problem with drinking. He was in constant conflict with his drinking and his political and religious convictions. There is a famous quotation about when he was in Rome teaching the Pantheon of the Gods to all of the aristocracy's children. The story goes that at night he would walk out into his garden, raise his arms up, look up towards the heavens, and say "God help me, but not yet." This seems to be an early version of the book we make reference to: *I'll Quit Tomorrow* by Dr. Vernon Johnson.

The attitude and the conflict between the fundamentalist and the definition of what constitutes grape juice and wine has been raised since the Protestant Reformation. I cited earlier the very neutral attitude on this subject. For example, biblically Christ demonstrates the value of wine in the marriage feast at Cana when he converts water into wine. Subsequent to that at the Last Supper he consecrates the wine and it becomes the basis for the Catholic's belief in Transubstantiation. The earlier Protestant Reformation group during the prohibition used St. Paul's letter to the Corinthians in which he says "Nor thieves, nor covetous, nor *drunkards*, nor revilers, nor extortioners, shall inherit the kingdom of God." 1 Corinthians 6:10 as the basis for not drinking wine.

Still today there is a conflict between the definition of grape juice and wine. The dispute revolves around the term "wine" in the Bible and the absence of the term "grape juice". The natural process for grapes is to quickly ferment into wine.

The name Carry Nation personifies the anger promoted by the temperance/prohibitionist movement. In the early 1900's, Carry Nation would destroy all of the liquor in a bar with her hatchet. This movement ultimately led to the passage of the Prohibition Act in 1919. Prohibition was unsuccessful because of public opposition and economic costs in lost taxes. There is a parallel in modern society about the debate over legalization of marijuana which will be discussed in a later chapter on drugs. The Prohibition Act (Volstead Act) was revoked in 1933.

Gin

The third major game changer occurred when the Dutch perfected the distillation of gin in the 17th century. A major change had to do with the development of the process of distillation. This was done by Dutch chemist Dr. Franciscus Sylvius who was able to create the distillation of gin to increase its alcohol content into the 40-50 percentile by a process of cooking and steam evaporation. The Italians were the first to develop gin but historically the Dutch are given credit for the abuse of it.

Gin was developed originally as a medicine to take care of certain medical problems, stomach problems primarily, and this was done with the use of botanicals. An article in Thought Catalog lists a few medicinal uses for gin. It is an antioxidant which can prevent cancer, increases cologen in skin, improves the digestive system (by the use of the juniper berry) and can be used as a natural remedy for arthritis.

By comparison, beer has an alcoholic content on average of approximately five percent by volume and wine approximately nine to sixteen percent. Gin on the other hand has an alcoholic content in excess of thirty seven percent by volume.

The history of Gin goes back to the 1600's where an article by the Oxford Group documented what is referred to as the Great Gin Epidemic. This epidemic took place in England in the late 1600's and early 1700's reaching its peak in 1750. One of the precursors of this so called epidemic was the Industrial Revolution which required workers to re- locate from the rural areas to the cities creating a totally new environment.

The development of gin coincided with the industrial revolution. There was a controlling philosophy at this time primarily espoused by Malthus, a statistician, who is famous for his work on world populations, which said that there were two types of populations. The inferior population, in this case the worker, and the genteel population which was the aristocracy. The purpose of the inferiors were to serve the government and the aristocracy. The population that was providing these physical services in this new workforce were a combination of adults, both men and women, as well as children. Later on this concept of using children in the workforce was carried out in the United States and was referred to as "sweat shops". The pay of these workers, adults and children alike, was partly in money and partly in gin. Gin was given on a weekly basis for the workers. This created some new problems since these workers were not accustomed to such a high alcoholic content. Many of the people referred to gin as "liquid madness". By the year 1750 the gin consumption exceeded three times that of the beer consumption in England.

There were attitudinal causes that were at work during this time also. As mentioned earlier was Malthus's concept about the inferior group being created simply for the use of government and the genteel populace. The second was the criticism of the workers because of the drunkenness, and the social problems associated with drunkenness, in the workforce. This attitude maintained that the inferiors (workers) were creating problems by the use of the alcohol even though the employer used gin as part of their pay.

During the Thirty Years War, gin was given to the troops before battle and this became known as "Dutch Courage". When the troops came home it became the favorite drink of the poor. The Gin Act was passed in an attempt to limit the amount of gin that was available by increasing its cost. Like its counterpart in the United States this became their "Prohibition". Since the poor people were the ones that were primarily the consumers of this liquid, there were riots in the streets. So the act which was passed in 1736 was later repealed in 1742.

There was a constant economic competition between the beer shops and the gin shops. This culminated ultimately in legislation limiting the way gin could be distributed. The people would not have the same freedom with gin that beer enjoyed.

The world-wide development of alcoholic beverages has taken on a nationalistic pride. Germans take pride in beer, the Dutch in gin, the word Scotch identifies Scotland, Vodka is Russian, Tequila is Mexican, wine is French, and bourbon the United States. The French take such pride in their wine that "new wine" is declared a national holiday called "Beaujolais Nouveau Day."

The attitude towards alcohol (beer, wine, or hard liquor) effects how people respond to a person who is alcoholic. Is alcoholism a disease or a moral issue? Your attitude will determine how you treat the alcoholic. It also requires a working knowledge of signs, symptoms, etiology, pathology, and prognosis of this illness.

CHAPTER 5

GRAPERS, INEBRIATES, ALCOHOLICS, AND SUBSTANCE ABUSERS

This chapter will be a reflection of society's attitude on the use of alcohol and the addiction to alcohol. It will also lay the foundation for the diagnosis and treatment of alcoholism. Some of the material may appear repetitious but I think it's important for the foundation of this chapter.

Earlier we described the term "graper" for someone who abused alcohol. Over the years in an attempt to describe the alcoholic, there have been other titles assigned to this condition or person. One that was very prominent in the late 1700's, early 1800's was the "inebriate". In 1830 Dr. Samuel Woodward called for the creation of inebriate asylums, the first of which opened its doors in 1864 in the state of New York. In 1870 the American Association for the Cure of Inebriety was founded under the principle that "inebriety was a disease".

This term "inebriate" stayed in use until around 1925. During this time period, inebriate asylums gave way to more private sanitariums called "jitter joints", "jag farms" or "dip shops". These were drying out farms where a person was taken off the alcohol but nothing was done to actually treat the long term conditions or effect of the illness.

During this same time period (1800's) alcoholism, unknown by that title, was considered to be a criminal offense and the best solution was to lock up individuals in a prison or some sort of mental institution and basically throw away the key. Unfortunately, many law enforcement organizations and legislators still think this is a solution to a medical problem.

Also in the 1840's there was an organization called the Washingtonians that promoted the idea of abstinence based on group dynamics. This was a very successful group of people, with a membership of approximately 500,000, practicing abstinence and was the precursor to AA.

Two things happened to destroy the Washingtonians and the value of the concept of abstinance. One was that the membership was divided on prohibition which was an issue in the 1800's and secondly, on slavery. Both of these were so controversial as to destroy its membership, and became the foundation for AA's principle that said "we never involve ourselves in any political or outside activities, our only purpose is to help the suffering alcoholic stay sober."

The first known use of the term "alcoholism" was in 1849 by a Swedish physician, Magnus Huss, who describes a disease resulting from chronic alcohol consumption and christens it "Alcoholismus chronicus". Alcoholism and the subsequent treatment of this condition took on varying forms over the next 200 years. Interventions ranged from water cures and mandatory sterilization to aversion therapies.

Over the years there has been a gradual change in the attitude towards the alcoholic as we begin to see many more attempts at institutional or private treatment for this condition. In 1879 Dr. Leslie Keeley announces "drunkeness is a disease and I can cure it". This resulted in about 200 Keeley Institute clinics located around the world. During the 20th century there was growing evidence and support for the idea that this was an illness and should be treated as such.

In 1935 we saw the first introduction of aversion therapy with the opening of the Shadel Sanatorium. This program was based on the aversion therapy concept which is "a person would drink, get intoxicated, or just before intoxication, would be required to vomit the contents of their stomach". There was actually a room in the treatment center called a vomitorium, in which this process was executed.

One of the greatest concepts in the treatment of alcoholism also occurred in 1935 when Bill Wilson, a stock broker, and Dr. Bob Smith, a physician, met in Akron, Ohio and founded the organization of Alcoholics Anonymous. The term AA was not used generally until 1939 when the Big Book was published under the name of Alcoholics Anonymous. So AA was not named after the organization but the organization was named after the Big Book of Alcoholics Anonymous.

Interestingly there was a number of people within the early AA organization that did not call themselves by that name. One that stands out in my mind was one of the more committed 12 steppers who would literally raid barrooms and drag people off to meetings. His group was called The Flying Squadron for the Rescue of Helpless, Hopeless Inebriates. In 1941 the Saturday Evening Post published an article on the fledgling movement of AA. Once that publication went national AA expanded exponentially all over the United States.

In the late 1930's and early 1940's there was a growing interest in the establishment of treatment programs to deal with alcoholism. Some of these early treatment programs were state facilities that were funded by public money and primarily managed by psychiatrists that were interested in the illness of addiction.

Most of these psychiatrists subsequently laid the foundation for the organization known as ASAM (American Society of Addiction Medicine).

Some of the names in the 1940's that were in the successful early treatment of alcoholism were Hazelden and St. Mary's, both located in Minnesota, and here in Baton Rouge, the chemical dependency unit of the Baton Rouge General Hospital (CDU), which gained national prominence as well.

In an attempt to establish a customary length of stay for treatment centers the following story is offered as an interesting aside as documented in the dialogue between a legislator and the administrators of the Hazelden Foundation in Center City, Minnesota.

The legislator, who was introducing a bill that required mandated services for alcoholism in health insurance in Minnesota, was looking for guidance on how long to document that treatment would be necessary. He called Hazelden and asked that question, and they said "It ranged anywhere from 5 to 7 to 10 days of detox, some people left at that time, other people stayed on for 20, 30, 40, days. So the legislator said "would 28 days be about average" and the agreement was "well yes I guess so" and so 28 days became the quote "medical model" for the length of time that a patient needed to be in treatment. There is no medical or scientific evidence to document anything other than it was a best guess.

During the early to mid 1940's we see companies such as Kaiser and Dupont implementing the first modern industrial alcoholism programs, which were the forerunners of today's employee assistance programs.

In 1944 Marty Mann founds the organization called the National Committee for Education of Alcoholism. This organization was founded on the following propositions:

> Alcoholism is a disease
> The alcoholic therefore is a sick person
> The alcoholic can be helped
> The alcoholic is worth helping

Beginning in the late 1940's and 50's we begin to see faith based programs emerge for the treatment of alcoholism. Al-Anon is established to provide support for family members whose life may be affected by an alcoholic family member or friend in 1951.

In 1952 the American Medical Association first defines alcoholism. In 1956 the American Medical Association stops short of declaring alcoholism a disease but does recognize alcoholics as legitimate patients.

The first important development in the 1960's occurred when E.M. Jellinek, known for the Jellinek bell curve, published *The Disease Concept of Alcoholism*. In the mid 1960's the insurance industry begins to reimburse the treatment of alcoholism on par with the treatment of other illnesses. In 1966 two federal Appeals Court decisions support the disease concept of alcoholism. The term "disease concept" is used only to describe the illness of alcoholism. Nowhere else is it used to describe an illness. One of the barriers of accepting alcoholism as a true illness is to diminish the term using disease concept. We do not call cancer the cancer concept or diabetes, the diabetes concept or other illnesses with that precursor. In 1967 the American Medical Association passes a resolution identifying alcoholism as a "complex" disease.

National attention was brought to this issue when Congress passed the Comprehensive Drug Abuse Prevention and Control Act in 1970. Also referred to as the Hughes Act, this was a major milestone in the nation's efforts to deal with alcohol abuse and alcoholism.

In 1971 The American Journal of Psychiatry published the "Criteria for the Diagnosis of Alcoholism". Also in 1971 alcoholism got a strong boost when it was recognized as being an occupational and health problem on the West Coast. With the formation of ALMACA (Association of Labor Management Consultants on Alcoholism) the workplace became the focus to deal with this problem. Today this organization is known as the Employee Assistant Professionals Association. The mid 1970's show the emergence of credentialing for counselors working in alcohol and drug treatment programs, and First Lady Betty Ford talks about her recovery from alcohol and drug addiction.

In spite of a long history dating back to the Greeks, Romans, and Magnus Huss, plus all subsequent legislation and treatment modes, we still have not come to grips accepting alcoholism as a disease.

A major setback to the treatment modality of alcoholism was the Patton State Hospital study. Another aversion therapy approach which was one of the gross experiments that was done on the re-introduction of the alcoholic to societal drinking was carried out at the Patton State Hospital in California in 1970.

This program was funded by the Addiction Research Foundation to document this concept. It was the theory of a husband and wife psychologist team, Mark and Linda Sobell, that alcoholics could be retrained to drink socially. The study involved 70 veterans since this was a VA Hospital, which were selected for their history of alcoholism. These veterans were split into two groups, half to a "controlled drinking" group and the other half to an "abstinence goal" group. Over a period of two years they were exposed to a form of aversion therapy with electric shock. At the end of the two years the experiment was reported as a total success.

Subsequently, one of the patients in that experiment got a copy of that report and began to check with his fellow veterans; as it turned out there was not one of the 34 remaining from the control group, one had died previously, that were social drinkers. When the information became public, one of the questions asked of him was "why do you think it did not work when you were discharged from the hospital? His comment was a very curt "I don't frequent bars where somebody is going to stick me with an electric prod after I have a couple of drinks".

In 1982, Pendery, Maltzman and West published an article, based on a ten year follow-up with subjects of this study, states that "a review of the evidence, including official records and new interviews, reveals that most subjects trained to do controlled drinking failed from the outset to drink safely." In a subsequent article, Maltzman is quoted as saying "beyond any reasonable doubt it's fraud." Because this was such a high profile case, there were contradictory reports on the Sobell studies. This was an embarrassment to the funding agency and if the consensus report of fraud was accepted there had to be a refund of the $750,000 grant money. Unfortunately, the critical documentation of this report is not always shown in the materials of university psychology departments.

There is also a theory of harm reduction, which says the patient is not ready to be totally abstinent, but that you can reduce the ingestion of alcohol, the number of times they will get drunk, on a harm reduction basis. The criteria is that if a patient was drinking seven days a week now they are only drinking and getting drunk two days a week. This creates a serious problem for some individuals who may work in an environment where there is a requirement by their employment of being totally abstinent or being without abusing of alcohol, while on the job. This is not an acceptable form of treatment. In particular for those that are under the jurisdiction and authority of the federal government and The Alcohol and Drugs in the Workplace Act, i.e. Coast Guard, DOT, Airlines, etc. That particular type of approach isn't practical from the point of view where total abstinence at the work site is required.

Fast forward from the 30's and 40's to the 80's and 90's where every treatment center was either a mental health provider or an alcoholism provider. Gradually there began to be a change in that position for two reasons. One, was the so called mental health parity bill, which excluded alcoholism from health insurance coverages but approved 45 days of in-patient mental health. Prior to that time we saw only the two definitions in the national utilization of the evaluation of patients, that of mental health or substance abuse and never the term behavioral health. The second, facilities were not paid or limited to a small detox time. It is during this time that we see increasing use of terms such as co-morbid or dual diagnosis.

Our own company, Health Associates of America, was a large utilization review company. Over a period of about 21 years we evaluated appropriateness of inpatient services based on diagnosis, treatment, and length of stay. Of those 17,000 reviews, both from a commercial point of view, an HMO, and from the federal government's coverage of substance abuse, the following information is submitted. As said we did not see any use of the term co-morbid condition or dual diagnosis until the late 1990's and early 2000's. Once that happened we began to see a change in statistics. Based on those 17,000 cases up until 2004, the accurate documentation for a dual diagnosis was less than about 12% to 15%. The reason that this is important is that we have seen a shift in the treatment of people with a dual diagnosis or co-morbid condition diagnosis.

The idea behind the dual diagnosis is that you want to make sure that you cover all the issues that maybe existing rather than focusing on a single issue such as mental health or substance abuse. In the attempt to do that these numbers have been skewed to as many as 70% to 80% of the people have a dual diagnosis and as a result the treatment and reimbursements have been predicated on those combination of services. Again the question is "follow the money, what's the best diagnosis for the best reimbursement?

If this new approach gave us a better outcome, then there could be some justification for the treatment going in this direction, however, evidence does not indicate that it gives a better outcome.

When I went to treatment in 1975 the cost on a per day basis, which was not covered by my health insurance by the way, was $75.00 a day. In 2017 that same type of service on a per diem basis would be somewhere between $1000.00 and $1250.00 per day. Again I raise the issue if the outcomes were better there might some kind of justification for the price increases.

The recovery rate in the 1950's and 60's as documented by ongoing follow-up with patients, was reported that about 50% of the people recovered from alcoholism. This meant that they did not go back to the use of alcohol and were totally abstinent. Of the additional 50% that did relapse, within several years following the relapse it dawned on them that maybe this was what they were told about it being a chronic illness, and so they went back to AA. Ultimately the numbers ranged anywhere from 60% to 75% that could be considered to be successful outcomes of abstinent treatment.

Today, that number according to the treatment centers themselves, the ones that keep valid numbers, and what SAMHSA numbers look like is somewhere around 20% to 25%, and that would be a high recovery rate. Bear in mind that alcoholism is a chronic illness and there is an expectation that there will be some problems in relapse. It has also been my experience and many others that are not associated with any treatment centers that the more bells and whistles you tie in to the program, i.e. aromatherapy, yoga, or poetry, lessens the recovery rate. This is not an indictment of the west coast but there is a common denominator which says that if you go to treatment in California you are going to get treatment with a view, but pay a price for the view as much out of proportion to what the services are worth.

With the requirement that substance abuse including alcoholism was covered under the Obama Health Care Plan, there was a proliferation of interest and money to go into the purchase and establishment of treatment centers.

These treatment centers and out- patient services range all the way from the use of the 12 Step program of Alcoholics Anonymous, which seems to be the common denominator for the success of in-patient and out-patient treatment programs. However, there are a number of critics of the 12 Step program that maintain that alcoholism is not a chronic illness, not an illness at all, and therefore should not be treated as such.

Many books have been written that say alcoholism is not a disease and therefore you can be retaught how to drink. This kind of thinking ranges from alcoholism is not a disease all the way to alcoholism being caused by a learning disability. In addition there are many programs that provide services to alcoholics which are referred to as "faith based" programs. These do not use the principles of AA with the exception that both have a belief in a higher power or in the case of faith based churches, a belief in Jesus Christ as the foundation of this service. There are no valid statistics to demonstrate the success of faith based programs to maintain abstinence.

Another criticism of the use of the AA approach is that there is no scientific definition or monitoring of the membership. Therefore membership in AA is not a valid form of recovery. AA has never maintained that it is a form of treatment. It is a self- help group by definition "one alcoholic helping another alcoholic to stay sober".

I challenge the critics of AA that say they have no valid recovery rate based on my own case. I attended my first AA meeting in March 1963, I did not get sober until December 1975. During that time I periodically attended AA. I think over time that many of the principles and concepts of recovery became an ingrained understanding of where I had to go. So my questions to the critics are "how do you give me credit? Are you saying that for all those years I attended meetings it did not work and how do you explain 41 years of sobriety based on the use of AA's 12 step program.

There is a new way of approaching treatment these days and that is to use a Medication Assisted Treatment (MAT) program in conjunction with other traditional treatment. Basically it says instead of the old system of blockers there is another drug on the market that can be used in the treatment of alcoholism. About 25 years ago that drug was called Naltrexone. Naltrexone is still in use and serves as a blocker to help cut down on the cravings. I had one patient, a physician that it was effective with, but that was one of the few that I saw its effectiveness.

The major changes in more recent times with MAT's is with the increase use of heroin. Heroin is an exponentially expanding drug problem in the country today. If nothing else the attention given to heroin and the overdoses caused by it, has been to create a moral sense of awareness to the problem of drugs and alcohol. In the case of heroin, there are two drugs that are used, one is methadone, which is the more traditional way, and has been on the market for a number of years, and has been effective in controlling cravings. One of the criticisms of Methadone is that once you are on it, you cannot get off of it. That is not necessarily true. A number of Methadone treatment centers do attempt to get their patients off of this drug, however there is a comparison between how to treat the heroin addict with the use of methadone and those who are on some sort of a maintenance program for Diabetes.

The second drug and newest kid on the block is Suboxone. This drug came on the market about 15 or 20 years ago. My first and only real successful experience with Suboxone was with a physician I had put into treatment four or five times. He reported to me that the first time he had constant cravings, even after all the treatment centers he attended. He said that once he got on Suboxone the cravings disappeared completely. Today he is completely restored back to his practice and is married and has a family. In this instance Suboxone has really been a life saver for him.

The difference between Methadone and Suboxone is that Methadone may be dispensed under the supervision of a nurse. Suboxone can only be dispensed under the supervision of a physician. The comparison between costs for Methadone treatment is about $400.00 a month as compared to about $1500.00 a month for Suboxone. It looks like the camel has its nose under the tent in the case of treatment for alcoholism or drug addiction in the advent of Suboxone and pharmaceuticals to treat addiction.

By way of introduction to the diagnostic portion of this history, let me comment on something that happened with my cardiologist. On a recent visit he asked if I would accept referrals from this clinic, there are approximately 50 cardiologists at the clinic. I laughed and said "yes but by the time you guys figure out if a patient has an alcohol or drug problem they are just this side of being dead." "What do you mean by that" he replied. "It's simple you all are trained in recognition of medical symptoms, i.e. the liver is enlarged, high blood pressure, cardiovascular problem, or there is some cognitive impairment all of which are some type of medical symptomologies. Those are late stage diagnostic pieces for alcohol and drugs. The early stages are all behavioral. I don't know of many physicians that are trained in recognition of addiction in the early stages."

I have been fortunate to study under three of the best teachers that I know in diagnosis. The first, Dr. Jon Weinberg and the second, Dr. Richard Heilman, were recognized in Chapter 2. The third was Dr. Louis Cataldie here in Baton Rouge. Dr. Cataldie has been one of the earliest physicians providing services to the alcoholic/addict. His experience and commitment is told in his book, *Coroners Journal*, describing treatment of some 20,000 alcohol/addict patients. He was one of the early developers of ASAM (American Society of Addiction Medicine) in Louisiana. He and I have worked in collaboration on some complex detoxification cases. Dr. Cataldie continues even today to educate his medical colleagues on addiction as a disease. I am very fortunate to have studied under and been associated with these three individuals.

Are you qualified to provide services for the alcoholic? Does your education and experience qualify you ethically and clinically in this field? What is your attitude toward the alcoholic and alcoholism? Do you have a bias on the question of depression vs addiction?

All of these are questions that led up to the need for clinicians to have a special license in addiction. There are four major disciplines in mental health: psychologists, social workers, licensed professional counselors, and licensed marriage and family therapists. Unfortunately, most doctoral and master degree programs do not have any specific education in addiction. Until recently physicians, and in particular psychiatrists, were not required or offered any courses in addiction in medical school. The failure of the higher education system to recognize the need for education and training in addiction totally ignores the statistic that 10% of the population suffers from addiction (SAMHSA).

With this background the Louisiana Association of Substance Abuse Counselors in Training (LASACT) introduced legislation to license addiction counselors in 1981. I have been a lobbyist representing the insurance agents, treatment providers, and alcoholism counselors since 1955. Because of my experience and personal interest in addiction, I was the lead lobbyist on this legislation.

Opposition came from every mental health profession. The oppositional argument was (1) we had no higher academic education/training and (2) there was no credited license examination. In response to these concerns it was pointed out that the universities offered very limited, if any, education in this field. Therefore, LASACT established its own academically qualified educational school in substance abuse. The curriculum on addiction is comprehensive in course content. It teaches that alcoholism is a primary, chronic, progressive, and terminal disease. It has its own pathology, symptomatology, and prognosis, which includes behavioral and medical symptoms. It is unlike any other disease. It also teaches that to be a substance abuse counselor you need knowledge, and an understanding of, pharmacology, basic anatomy and physiology, psychology, and multiple counseling theories (Adlerian, Existential, Humanism, Cognitive, Gestalt, Behaviorism, Transactional Analysis, Reality Therapy, and Family Systems). Upon completion, the student will have earned 180 hours of academic training specific to addiction as required by the Louisiana State Statute for Licensure.

To address the second oppositional concern, an oral and written exam, was offered for candidates seeking licensure. This exam was based on the national and international accepted criteria of the ICRC (International Certification & Reciprocity Consortium).

The following story illustrates the need for this certification/licensure. I was called as an expert witness in a divorce case. I had attempted an intervention on the plaintiff. In the middle of the intervention, the identified alcoholic bolted from the room and contacted his attorney. His attorney advised him to seek a full medical and psychological evaluation, which he subsequently did. This leading to my appearance in the courtroom. Now the typical exchange between opposing counsels is to determine if the proposed expert witness is qualified to be an "expert".

I have testified as an expert witness in 14 cases. I was on the stand, in this case, a total of 6 hours, longer than any other case. At the time of this particular case we did not have certification/licensure in the addiction field. After several hours of cross-examination, the opposing counsel said "Mr. Hidalgo, it appears that you are not certified in this field by licensure. What you have done, is you and someone like you in your field, examine each other and then say you are certified to practice in this field." My response was "counselor that's about right and we took this concept from lawyers. Let me explain-years ago I could have come to you and said I would like to work with you as a law clerk instead of going to law school. After 4 or 5 years as your clerk, you'd say to me, Don, I think you know enough about the law to hang out your shingle and practice with me. So counselor, if that system is good enough for lawyers, it's good enough for us." At this point the Judge approved me as an expert.

Further questioning went like this, "Mr. Hidalgo, would you say that Ochsner Hospital is qualified to do a psychological and medical evaluation on alcoholism? I respond "yes". "Mr. Hidalgo you raised the question about my client having chest pains and his EKG proved negative. How do you explain this?" I turn to the Judge and say "you qualified me as an expert witness in the field of addiction, opposing counsel requires an opinion medically, may I answer it?" The Judges comment was "he opened this can of worms and I want to hear the answer." I simply replied "that an EKG would not show the effect alcohol had on the heart. Alcohol will cause an inflammation of the myocardial lining of the heart, not picked up on an EKG." Opposing counsel then asked, "Mr. Hidalgo you accused my client of having a mental problem since he could not remember certain things. Are you telling this court that you have never had any little memory lapses." My response: "not since I quit drinking, counselor". It was obvious that he did not know about alcoholism or blackouts caused by alcoholism.

This story demonstrates the need for specific education and training in behavioral and medical problems to diagnose alcoholism. The first legislation for certification was introduced in 1981. It took us until 1988 to get certification for substance abuse counselors approved by the state of Louisiana. We did not achieve licensure until 2005. Today Louisiana is recognized as having one of the most comprehensive licensure laws on addiction. Under the title of licensure, the following addictions are covered: alcohol, drugs, sex, gambling, and eating disorders.

My experience has been, unless you have specific academic training in alcoholism/substance abuse as to signs and symptoms of behavior and medical problems, you cannot ask the right questions to form a diagnosis.

How do we diagnose alcoholism and drug addiction? First you have to establish the fact that there is a difference between abuse and addiction. Abuse is something that if a person gets drunk is prima fascia that they are alcoholic. It's not smart to do that but it's not a total indication they are alcoholic. It may be stupid but it's not alcoholism.

Once we have passed the point of the medical criteria then we are now into what we describe as addiction from a medical perspective. How do we go through this process? The questions that you need to ask are represented by the following: have you ever had anyone comment on your drinking? Have you ever had anyone to suggest you had a personality change, not for the better when you were drinking? Has anyone ever suggested to you that your personality changes from when you are drinking or not drinking? Has your spouse, family member, or friend ever commented that you are drinking too much? Be careful of this one because family members are pretty cautious about trying to address the issue for fear of some reaction from the alcoholic. However it is important to get some insight from the family perspective. Again, has your husband or wife, children, parents, brothers, and sisters commented that somehow you may be drinking too much or you made a fool of yourself at a recent get together? Do you always remember what is happening when you are drinking or are there times when you cannot recall pieces of the night before? The question you are leading up to there is the possibility of blackouts. Be careful how you do that, because many times people will recognize where you are going and they will deny that that happens. You do need to establish whether or not they have been impaired as a result of blackouts. One of the other questions I find very helpful is comparing their drinking to that of their peers –do you hold your alcohol as well as they do, less than they do, or more than they do? Men can be braggadocios and say I hold my liquor better than my peers do.

One of the symptoms of alcoholism is tolerance and tolerance means being able to hold your liquor better than your peers. The follow-up question to this is "have you noticed that it doesn't take as much to get you loaded as before?" That's an indication your tolerance is going down. On the other hand if it takes a little more that's an increase in tolerance. Either direction are indications that this needs to be explored.

I find that it is helpful to intersperse some medical related questions along with the behavioral pieces. Some examples of medical questions could be, "has a doctor ever told you that you have high blood pressure or if you have an enlarged liver? Have you ever complained about chest pains not associated with a heart condition? Behavioral questions could be, "are you having any difficulty in managing your money particularly after you've been drinking? Do you have difficulty in figuring out how you spent your money when you were drinking? Have you ever asked yourself would I be better off if I didn't drink or didn't drink so much? Has that thought ever occurred to you? This is indicative of self-disclosure or self-introspection.

Occupationally, you need to question if they had any problems on the job. Have you ever had any time you were unable to go to work because of your drinking? Have you ever been late for work because of your drinking? Have you ever had a problem performing at your best or normal level after having drank? Have you ever been disciplined by your employer because of your drinking? Have you ever tested positive for a drug or alcohol test?

If you are working with a young person in school, the questions should focus on scholastics. The occupation of the student is measured by class attendance and grades. A key question here is "have you ever dropped a subject because you do not attend enough classes or have you ever been on scholastic probation?"

Because most programs I recommend have a spiritual base, I try to establish early what the spiritual or religious background of the patient is. I do this by asking about their growing up years and if they had any kind of religious training. I do not ask them, at this time, where they are today in their religious views. This early questioning gives me an indication of where I may be able to go later on with respect to the question about their concept of God or what they believe, and that creates an opportunity to discuss if they feel okay with themselves in their relationship with a spiritual being.

Another question I find very effective is "have you ever felt that you were different than everyone else, that somehow you just didn't fit in?" or "have you ever felt that you were lonely without being alone?" There is a difference between being alone and lonely. Being lonely is an indication that alcohol is isolating the victim.

Remember that one of the common characteristics of alcoholism is a sophisticated denial system or a rationalization or justification of the answer they will give you. If you have established the criteria for determining if it is alcohol or drug addiction, then the next step is to figure out the most appropriate, cost effective, and least restrictive treatment program for your patient to attend.

Treatment options can range all the way from AA, an educational program, an in-patient program, or even out-patient programs. All of those are factors you need to become experienced with and know what treatment programs are available to be able to provide your clients with the most appropriate treatment.

I feel so strongly about counselors being qualified by experience and education to work in this addiction field, that we established an educational foundation in my wife's name when she died 19 years ago. She was the family counselor for a substance abuse treatment program and the family decided the best way to honor her memory would be to provide funding for an education program for counselors to help them achieve a master's level degree here in Louisiana and/or become licensed addiction counselors. Since its inception we have provided scholarship funds for over 200 counselors in training.

So how do you pick a treatment center? If you go on the website almost all treatment centers begin with the statement that we are a dual diagnosis program, we are prepared to offer you services for all kinds of problems. There are several national treatment centers that maintain most of the problems with alcohol, and the abuse of medications, stems from a traumatic event in a person's life. If you didn't have a traumatic event when you checked in they will find one for you before you check out.

Over the last 40 years we have established a criteria that determines the type of treatment programs used, or treatment approach used, based on the client's needs. However there are some common denominators that we look for; for instance, does the program use the 12 Steps as a basis for recovery? Does the program have a counseling staff that possess clinical licensure specifically in substance abuse not just a mental health license? Is the medical director an ASAM certified physician, whether he is an internist or a psychiatrist, he should be ASAM certified. I reference ASAM specifically because of my experience and relationship with Dr. Louis Cataldie, whom I consider to be one of the pre-eminent ASAM physicians in the United States, having treated over 20,000 patients himself.

If I refer a person to treatment, in-patient or out-patient, I want a weekly progress report to keep me informed of what is going on with the patient. I do not need to be involved in the treatment process but I do want to be kept informed about any problems that may arise since we are going to be responsible for the re- integration of the patient back into an aftercare program.

One of the most important pieces in our selection of a treatment program, is that it must have a strong family component. By that I mean there must be at least 4 or 5 days with the families at the treatment center, interacting with the patient a couple of hours during the sessions, otherwise we do not refer to those treatment facilities. Also we require that if we send a patient to treatment that the family commits to participating in family week as well. We know from experience that unless the family gets involved in the recovery process the odds of the patient recovering are slim to none.

Post services are equally as important as the primary treatment. The patient should be involved in AA on a weekly basis for the first 90 days and seeing a substance abuse counselor on a weekly basis or more frequently as needed.

There should also be couples counseling in conjunction with the individual counseling for the patient. I site these based on my experience with about

2000 patients of my own plus my own life experience in recovery. I am convinced that unless I had made arrangements for aftercare for my wife and I, and my children, I would not be in recovery today.

Despite all of this documentation of alcoholism being a complex disease; society, the medical community, and insurance companies do not treat it as such. Today there is no diagnosis of alcoholism. According to the DSM, it is a substance use disorder.

So what happened to the diagnostic term "alcoholism"? Some of the critics have cited that people feel stigmatized by this term. So what causes alcoholism specifically- it is the misuse or abuse of alcohol, not a substance in the abstract term.

If there is such a public opinion against the term alcoholism, why has AA continued to grow? Reported by the General Service Office, as of January 2016 there are 60,698 AA groups in the United States totaling 1,262,542 members. Worldwide there are 117,748 AA groups and 2,089,698 members.

I think this proves two things: AA is a viable, growing organization and there are millions of people who identify themselves as recovering alcoholics. So where is the stigmatization?

CHAPTER 6

EVOLUTION OF THE EMPLOYEE ASSISTANCE PROGRAM

The concept of dealing with personal, family, and occupational problems in the work setting using the EAP held great promise initially. Unfortunately it has not fulfilled its bright and shining original premise of using the workplace to remediate personal and occupational problems, for a number of reasons which will be presented in the following chapters.

Perhaps the first EAP had an Irish accent. In Stephen Mansfield's book *Of God and Guinness: Biography of the Beer that Changed the World* he documents that Arthur Guinness founded in effect what was the first EAP. Arthur Guinness recognized that there was a great value in having productive employees and as a result he established a program that provided counseling and health services for his employees. This was back in the 1700's.

As we move forward in history we find that there was a growing need on the part of business to deal with alcohol issues in the workplace. The early forerunners of this program were both political, business, and labor in nature. During the Richard Nixon administration, Senator Hughes, a recovering alcoholic himself, became the advocate and voice for a program to deal with alcoholism in the workplace. The concept of dealing with this in the workplace is very fundamental because it deals with two issues in the average person's life; the family and the paycheck. If you can establish a program that deals with both, you have the ideal vehicle to affect changes in the workplace environment.

In the early years the only people involved in the actual providing of services at the work site were recovering alcoholics themselves that were assigned to interview and help employees by referring them to resources in the community. These were strictly peer programs.

In the mid 1940's efforts at more formalized alcoholism programs were led by the Yale Center of Alcohol Studies. The Yale Plan for Business and Industry promoted a nine step plan for implementing an occupational alcoholism program. As you read the following, you will see that it is almost an exact description of what ALMACA adopted as being the core requirements for a successful EAP. Those nine steps were: 1)education of top management, 2)assignment of program responsibility to an existing department, 3)selection and training of a coordinator to administer the program, 4)mobilization of internal intervention resources, 5)development of a company-wide policy regarding relationship of treatment to discipline, 6)linkage to alcoholism treatment services, 7)supervisory training, 8)employee orientation and education, and 9) periodic surveys to assess the extent of the problem within the company (Henderson and Bacon, 1953).

The following is cited as an example of the limited scope of services viewed by the counseling community of an EAP. I was asked to give a presentation (3 hours duration) on EAP's at the International Social Worker's Conference. The title of the talk was "What is an EAP?" I asked the audience what their definition of an EAP was and the answer universally was a counseling program. I replied to this "If that's all an EAP is, then within 5 years I will be out of business. If it is way more than I described, most of you will be working for an EAP firm like mine."

When the EAP concept moved forward to a pilot basis, Occupational Program Consultants or OPC's were established in each state to organize occupational alcoholism programs in business and industry. These first OPC's became known as the Thundering 100. Rutgers University established a summer program to train these OPC counselors in the documentation and recognition of alcoholism in the workplace. I am proud to say that one of my staff who is now the director of our national and international affiliate program was one of the counselors trained at Rutgers University.

There is a question about who was the first company to actually adopt a working alcoholism program in the workplace. It ranges from Dupont, Eastman Kodak, Kennecott Copper Company and Allis Chalmers. The idea germinated and had such strong support that it began to pop up among a number of companies.

Alcoholics Anonymous also had an influence in this movement. On February 8, 1940, John D. Rockefeller called together a number of the top executives in the Unites States for a black tie dinner and gave the founders of AA, Dr. Bob Smith and Bill Wilson, an opportunity to explain what the new program of Alcoholics Anonymous was all about, how effective it was, and how it operated. Mr. Rockefeller recognized that this program had nothing to do with money, it had to do with one suffering alcoholic helping another suffering alcoholic and in so doing they both got into recovery. This became the genesis of the peer involvement in the alcoholism program and subsequently the EAP programs.

I'm afraid that we have lost sight of the importance and the value of using recovering individuals, who with training and their unique experience in recovery, in the EAP services.

Further in the book I will discuss how this program has changed dramatically over the years.

In Louisiana our former governor, Edwin Edwards, recognized the value of an occupational alcoholism program, and he issued Legislative Executive Order #74 (1974) which recommended that there be a state wide program adopted to deal with alcoholism. A group was called together to study and implement this program. I cite this because it is typical of what happened in EAPA later on. A committee under the direction of Ronald Falgoust, Deputy Director of Health and Human Services was created which included internal state employees, external providers, and human resources personnel. After about two years of discussion it was decided the state would implement a program and it would be administered on an external EAP basis. Unfortunately this program was never implemented as intended. There was a program ultimately adopted but it did not in any way resemble what we would describe as an EAP.

It was during the 1960's and 1970's that the real development of external EAP's caught fire. The following were the six earliest national external EAP's that we can document. Otto Jones, founder of International Affairs, documented the cost effectiveness (ROI) of an EAP. Bud Larsen, founder of Metropolitan Clinic Counseling was the pioneer of the concept of cost control using carve-outs. Robert Doer, developed the relationship with the Railroad Industry using EAP to deal with alcohol issues. Brownlee Dolan Stein, gave birth to the use of an affiliate counselors system to manage nationwide EAP's.

Performance Personnel Services, was originally a staffing provider for medical personnel and subsequently developed into an EAP. Hidalgo Health Associates, an early pioneer established strong relationships by providing manager training and employee orientation. The introduction of interventions with corporate personnel allowed HHA to demonstrate the economic value of retaining key employees. This resulted in an expansion of the business to national and international clients. Hidalgo Health Associates is the only one of the original group to still be in operation today.

All of us had a common interest in Family Counseling Services because they were marketing their EAP's as a nonprofit which gave them a major competitive advantage over us. This organization provided counseling services on a local community wide basis. The Xerox Corporation promoted the use of their services with a corporate donation. Family Counseling Services promoted their EAP to meet these match funds. Therefore, we agreed to hire a lobbyist in Washington, D.C. to remove their competitive advantage. This was subsequently done through the IRS.

As an indication of how serious this problem was, the following story is used to illustrate this point. We were invited by a corporate client to do a presentation on our services. The Family Counseling Services marketing representative emphasized their community service and nonprofit status. The corporate client officer asked me, "Are you also a nonprofit?" To which I replied, "Not intentionally."

At this point we need to define the two organizations dedicated to providing these services. Those organizations were ALMACA (Association of Labor Management Administrators and Consultants on Alcoholism) and then subsequently EAPA (Employee Assistance Professionals Association).

So who were the original founders of ALMACA? This organization founded in 1971, was a combination of labor and management coming together with a joint interest in providing services for the suffering alcoholic and at the same time providing an improvement in workplace performance on the part of its employees.

The concept of ALMACA originated on the West Coast among a group of businesses that were concerned about the impact that alcohol and alcoholism was having on the workplace, the expenses of health insurance and the lost productivity of the workforce. Two other organizations instrumental in the formation of this movement were the local councils on alcoholism and the NIAAA (National Institute on Alcoholism and Alcohol Abuse).

In spite of the fact that the title was the Association of Labor Management Administrators and Consultants on Alcoholism, labor was not initially a driving force in the formation of ALMACA. Labor was very cautious about joining or supporting this concept. Their great fear was that management would use this as a tool to bypass the arbitration and grievance procedures in place used to protect a union employee that had an alcohol problem. It was not until people like Wilbert Brant, a local Buffalo, New York, bus driver and labor representative, became involved in the local alcoholism programs because he saw the value of using joint strengths of labor and management to deal with workplace alcoholism problems, that the concept received support. Subsequently he went to Washington, D.C. as the National Council on Alcoholism's advocate to promote joint efforts between the AFL-CIO and NIAAA. Subsequently the AFL-CIO and the Stevedores Union became members in ALMACA.

One of the problems initially faced was that the local chapters on alcoholism viewed this new program as their imminent domain and resented the fact that they were external EAP's coming into the field and usurping their authority, responsibility, and income.

Great civilizations have destroyed themselves from within. The Greek cities destroyed their cultural and military might by in-fighting among themselves. The Romans, one of the greatest civilizations ever to exist, destroyed itself with corruption from the policies of the Senate. It destroyed the incentive of the people to work by providing free food and entertainment at the Coliseum Circus. Nikita Khruschev prophesized that the United States would destroy itself from within. He could foresee what we are experiencing in the United States today.

Based on this concept, it is amazing that ALMACA survived at all since they had so many divergent opinions, groups, fears, anxieties, and needs, all conflicting together to resolve itself into a single entity to address this workplace problem. It was not until the mid-1970's that ALMACA began to take form as to what it subsequently would become. I joined ALMACA in 1976 and attended my first ALMACA conference in Detroit shortly thereafter.

At this time I was involved in occupational alcoholism programs as I documented in my early history. I attended the conference in Detroit and was impressed with two things: the first being the commitment on the part of the membership to deal with alcoholism in the workplace and second how that was accomplished.

There were two people that stand out in my mind and in the history of ALMACA. One was John Hennessey, President of the Longshore Workman's Union in New York and subsequently years later George Cobb of the West Coast Stevedores Union. These two people impressed me with their commitment on the part of labor to support this program.

On an individual note, one of the meetings I attended during the Detroit conference was on Peer Reviews. The speaker at that meeting identified himself as Little Paul. Little Paul was a seaman who sailed between Boston and England routinely. He described on one occasion how a shipmate of his came aboard drunk and in the process of trying to sober him up, went into seizures and was experiencing DT's. Little Paul described how he and some of the other recovering alcoholics aboard ship sat with him and nursed him through that by "giving him a little of the hair of the dog that bit it", which meant they kept feeding him small amounts of alcohol to bring him through the detox. A mixture of honey, orange juice, and alcohol can also work in this situation. I doubt seriously that there are many recovering alcoholics let alone EAP counselors that have ever experienced the responsibility of trying to detox a person individually without medical assistance. I myself have been involved with this on a number of occasions, one of which I described in the plane trip returning home after having done an intervention on a physician.

One of the great strengths in the early history of ALMACA was the personal involvement of senior management. Many times the chief executive officers of major corporations expressed their personal support of the program. This is particularly true in my quote, given at the beginning of this book when I talked about the president of the Russell Corporation and the involvement that Gene Gwaltney and his wife Nancy, had in the formation of the EAP services. Their support for an EAP in their company had a great impact in the long term for our company as well as other companies. The message became clear to middle managers and senior managers that if the president was involved in the program than they also should be involved. Suffice it to say that it took a combination of senior management and middle management's involvement and personal attention to make this program as successful as it was in the 1970's and 80's.

So from 1971 until the early 80's and then in the late 80's there was a radical change in the EAP. At this time it is important that I point out one of the issues that I believe was a major contributor that caused a serious rift in EAP's.

There was a growing issue of professionalism within the ranks of the EAP which was in conflict with the concept of the peer support and peer review type of program. The two parties whom I know personally, who documented this was Dr. Paul Roman Ph.D. Dr. Roman, who at the time that I knew him, was a professor at Tulane University, now with the University of Georgia, and has been a great historical source for the history of EAP's. The second, Dr. Paul Tisher, University of Pennsylvania, also wrote many scholarly papers on alcoholism in the workplace documenting the effectiveness of workplace programs.

At this point there was a serious movement on how to change ALMACA from a peer provider service to a broad based mental health/alcoholism academic recognition. Perhaps one of the greatest sources of information to describe the attempt to go from a peer review program to a professional program are in the papers written by Dr. Paul Hufnagel, Ph.D., L.C.S.W.

In his papers and subsequent documentation on recommendations for the CEAP (Certified Employee Assistance Professional) certification, he goes into great detail to describe what the turning point was in the history of the ALMACA organization. He points out very, very, vividly the problem that almost caused the destruction of the ALMACA organization. His point was that there was a separation between two concepts of what a CEAP was, and stood for, Certified Employee Assistance Professional. The title states certified, it does not say licensed employee assistance professional. This is where the conflict came in.

ALMACA at its headquarters began to move away from the concept of a peer review or a non-licensed counselor by definition of CEAP to one that had to have at a minimum a master's degree or in some states even a Ph.D.

I am deeply grateful to Dr. Hufnagel for the assistance he gave me by providing the early writings on the potential problems to be faced in the CEAP program. I was part of the research group that helped document the information necessary for which I am grateful.

In 1982, I introduced a bill to the Louisiana legislature to certify employee assistance professionals. I had no idea at the time as a lobbyist, what a hornet's nest I was creating. Immediately I had opposition from the social workers, who alleged that this bill would prohibit them from providing EAP services. In one of the committee hearings, there was a social worker by the name of Billy April that testified "if this bill was passed the Hidalgo EAP police could have us arrested for practicing without a certificate as a CEAP." This comment was a master stroke that killed the bill in committee that year.

In addition I had opposition from the AFL-CIO because I had included one of their members on our board. I thought it was important to have a member from the labor group to be part of this process since they were one of the original founders of ALMACA. They declined to be appointed to the board. I also had recommended a representative of the human resource association to be a member on the board. I got a call from the HR association with three of their attorneys on the line threatening to sue me if I put their people on the board of CEAP's. Again I was surprised because I thought surely human resource people would recognize the value of an EAP and would want to be a part of that process. I took them out of the certification law.

The final death note of my bill was when I got a phone call from John Maynard, president of EAPA, telling me he was going to be in New Orleans and to meet him at Pascal Manale's Restaurant. Included in this meeting were members of the New Orleans EAPA chapter, mostly social workers, who had been adamantly opposed to this bill. That night at the restaurant John Maynard threatened to sue me personally and tell me I did not have the right to use the certification of employee assistance professionals in my legislation.

As further documentation of the problem, I received a phone call from the national EAPA headquarters legislative advisor, telling me that I would have to use their model bill in order to pass my legislation successfully. However, one of the problems in using their bill was that it contained punitive damages for violations of any of the practice acts. The business community of Louisiana is adamant about not having punitive damages. I was serving on the board of directors of LABI (Louisiana Association of Business and Industry) at the time. This organization is the largest group representing 80,000 large and small employers in Louisiana. They told me they would fight this bill, tooth and nail, if I kept the punitive damages piece in. I subsequently agreed to take it out. When I notified Washington what the final bill would look like I was accused of being a racist since the person who was behind the use of the EAPA bill, rather than my bill, was a black female counselor in New Orleans.

I have been in practice for a number of years and a number of my employees are black so I resented the hell out of someone saying I was racist. This bill was introduced in three different legislative sessions and each time I had to fight off opposition primarily from the social workers. Finally, I was able to get an agreement with the social workers and they backed off of the bill and it was passed, as a certification, not a licensure. Subsequently signed by the governor, the bill became law and confirmed the members of our board.

However, prior to our first board meeting, I experienced one of the most blatant political moves I have ever seen against my legislation. Someone, I always suspected the social workers of the New Orleans EAPA chapter, contacted a particular legislator who had a reputation for wiping out boards that had not been meeting. Since we had not had our first board meeting, the legislation creating the EAP certification was taken off the books.

There have been only two states to have successfully passed legislation regarding EAP licensure. At the present time North Carolina is the only state with licensure of EAP professionals but it requires the candidate to have an advanced degree. Tennessee originally had legislation passed but like us it became a certification. So at this stage, only one state out of fifty has been successful in passing EAP licensure.

You couple this internal battle of moving the position of ALMACA from a peer alcoholic program to a professional academic organization with an event that occurred at the 1988 convention in Baltimore. Leading up to this convention there had been some rumbling about discord between labor and management and what was happening with respect to ALMACA's board activity and where we were going. Labor felt that we were moving entirely in the direction of becoming an "academically licensed organization" as oppose to the idea of labor being involved at a peer support level.

So what happened at the 1988 convention, I can sum it up by telling you my experience at breakfast with the labor unions, which historically has always been one of the most interesting events of the ALMACA conferences. The breakfast would start with the local Marine Corps band coming in bringing the flag and the United States standard, playing the Star Spangled Banner, salute to the flag, and then an opening prayer.

I was seated at a table with members of the United Auto Workers Union-Ford Division, when one of them turned to me and asked "What happened to our EAP program? What is going on here? There is no room for us anymore in what's happening. What do we do?" I looked at him and felt that I did not have an answer for his questions because I sympathized with him and unfortunately saw the same thing that he saw but from perhaps a different perspective.

The program at that conference took on an entirely different approach as far as the purpose and value of ALMACA. It was at that conference that several things occurred:

(1) There had been a recommendation to change the name from AL-MACA to EAPA. EAPA being the most appropriate definition of who we were. There was a lot of opposition to the change in name but also what the intent of the change meant. Unfortunately those that had concerns about the change were accurate in their fears.

(2) What we saw at that convention was that most of the presenters were academicians coming from universities. Most of the presentations were based on what the "studies" said we should be doing rather than what had worked for us on a practical basis.

(3) There was a strong presence on the part of health insurance plans. Their proposal, based on studies which indicated that the best approach for using EAP's was the use of health insurance companies, to provide these services. It was at this point that health insurance companies captured the EAP field and turned it into something that was an insurance product rather than what the EAP's intended. How did they do this? They said "if you buy our health insurance we will give you a free EAP." What does free mean? Does it truly mean that something is provided without any cost upfront or later on? The question is answered very simply –there is no such thing as free. There has to be compensation somewhere. So in the case of the insurance companies it was buy our insurance and we will give you this program.

In the use of "free" EAP services you are guaranteed that you are going to have an insurance claim because you cannot resolve many problems within the three session model. Just to clarify, an insurance EAP was limited to three sessions and those sessions could come in the form of a website visit or telephone call. So what often happens is that the counselor that is contracted with the insurance company says, near the end of the second or third session, "sorry I can't provide you any more "free" services under the EAP insurance contract however I can move you over to my private practice and now I can continue to provide these services and I will bill your insurance company." The transition between free EAPs and now billing is where the real trap is. There is generally no understanding by the insured about how this happened and who is really paying for the EAP services. We have documented on a number of occasions how this bait and switch program has cost the companies millions of dollars in the "free" EAP programs.

So what happened in 1988? We saw several things occur that almost destroyed this movement. The change in name, the implication of what that meant, the philosophical differences between labor and management, labor subsequently withdrawing from the organization, the advent of the insurance companies and the concept of a licensed person to provide EAP services. In describing the withdrawal of the labor unions from the association it was almost like the spirit of the alcoholism and the early days that created this program were completely sucked out of EAPA and now we became just another mental health provider organization.

Let me go back to my original premise in the opening paragraph, are we about to destroy a great organization by this internal conflict. I strongly suggest that EAPA take a look at its position on its intent and how it has affected the provider community. The concept of the CEAP was promoted by EAPA. It was promoted with great enthusiasm, and an intent to publicize the value of that certification, so that most companies would see the value and hire a CEAP or that most request for services (RFP) would document the value of a CEAP on the provider staff. I personally never saw the real commitment to promoting CEAP services. At least not in the concept that was acceptable to the community itself, not in the academician sense.

As evidence of this I would ask EAPA to advise how many people are really CEAP's or have earned the CEAP certification compared with the total number of members in the association itself. In line with this I have asked at a number of EAPA conferences and our state wide association meetings the following question-"What is your primary license and your service?" Very few will tell you that their primary service is EAP. They will tell you what their license is –"I am a LPC, LCSW, I'm a marriage and family counselor, I'm a psychologist," but they won't tell you that their primary interest is in EAP. That in itself tells me what part of the problem is. EAPA and the associations have not done a good job on promoting the value to the individual practitioner of what that certification means.

In January of this year we saw a major change in the administration and leadership of EAPA with the appointment of Greg DeLapp. I personally contacted Mr. DeLapp and have spoken about the history of the EAP and to gain insight into his appreciation of this profession. He worked as an EAP coordinator for the Champion Corporation for many years which gives him a good perspective as a practitioner of what the problems are. I sincerely hope his leadership will change us in the right direction.

I consider my primary occupation to be that of an alcoholism administrator as well as a licensed addiction counselor providing personal EAP services in the traditions that founded this organization. As I have said previously I have been a member since 1976 and it is my hope that as my career comes to a close that we will see a regeneration in the enthusiasm for EAPA internally as well as externally.

Have all of these changes added to your interest in providing EAP services? Has it given your patient/client an improved quality of life or better outcome? Will it add to your income and practice?

CHAPTER 7

NOT MY JOB

If you have ever said "that's not my job" you may have just stopped learning and growing your practice. One expression that was not acceptable in our company was for a person to say, when they were asked to do something, "that's not my job". Now it may not be my job, but if it's a request that needs to be met by one of our clients or patients, and if we don't have the skills to be able to do it, then we need to find someone else in the organization or go outside the organization to meet that client's needs.

As I said at the beginning of this book, I would be giving you some citations of some unusual and outstanding characteristics of the development of EAP services as a result of our relationship with the Russell Corporation.

We had been in operation and providing EAP services for approximately three years prior to the time we took on the Russell Corporation account. We had already developed a pretty sophisticated training program for supervisors as well as orientation for the employees. In addition we had put together a multi-discipline staff to meet the typical types of problems that presented in an EAP setting. The Russell Corporation had some 13,000 employees scattered over a seven state area. They were primarily in the textile business, making and manufacturing T-shirts and athletic uniforms, as a matter of fact they were called the Russell Athletic Company.

When I met with the president, Gene Gwaltney, and explained to him what I needed with respect to time from his supervisors, which meant time to train them on how to be good supervisors, and when and how and under what circumstances to refer people to the EAP, he looked at me and said "you want my people for seven hours, that's an entire work day." I said "that's correct" and he replied, "do you have any idea what kind of costs you are talking about to pull my people off line." I replied "it's going to cost you approximately $12 million if you decide to do this." He looked at me quizzically and said "how did you figure that?" It's simple, "I know what your supervisors make and multiply that times the 3000 supervisors that will be involved in this program." "So why should we do that, he questioned. Well, let's put it this way, you are going to pay me the same whether I see one of your 13,000 employees or I see all 13,000 of them, so it's up to you, do you want to get the most for your money? If you give us the opportunity to make sure that your first line supervisors truly understand the value to them personally of what we are doing and why you are doing it, then you need to give me that much time." So to his credit, he agreed to do it. It took us about 7 months to complete the entire training program for the supervisors.

The training program itself was divided into three sections: first, it was designed to help the supervisor have a fundamental understanding of signs and symptoms of impairment as a result of addiction.

Second, it was designed to help the supervisor to understand a little about human psychology. We had a manual that had been compiled, copyrighted, and published in connection with the professor of psychology at LSU, Dr. Edwin Timmons.

I met Dr. Timmons when he was doing psychological services for the business administration program at LSU. Dr. Timmons was fascinated with the concept that an EAP could serve a great purpose as far as improving the profitability and manageability of problem employees in the work setting. As a matter of fact I lectured the MBA class at LSU on the values of, and how an EAP would work, through the strength and recommendation of Dr. Timmons. As a result of these lectures we were selected to provide the EAP services to LSU's 11,000 faculty and employees. When Dr. Timmons retired, I hired him as a consultant to come in and help us develop this manual I am describing now. The section on what the supervisor needed to know about human psychology was titled "Behavioral Dynamics". There is an analogy used in that section that many years later people would come up to me and say "I remember the onion skinned concept", which told me they really had listened to this seven hour program we were presenting.

The third part of the training program, represented by the last section of the manual, was designed specifically to help the supervisor have a degree of comfort with understanding on what to expect and how to deal with the obstacles of an employee questioning whether or not it was appropriate or why they needed to see the EAP.

As a result of the management training programs the normal referral rate at that time would be around 5% of the employee population. In the Russell Corporation's case it exceeded 10% to 15% in some instances. It was not solely on the supervisors making referrals but it was with a deep and accepting understanding of the opportunity to deal with problems in the employee workforce.

Because we were working in a primarily rural area there was no opportunity to establish individual offices, therefore we had what we referred to as the "milk run", and we actually went to the sewing machine sites and had an opportunity to counsel with the employees there. On occasion we were given the manager's office to conduct our services. In any event the employees would sign up to let us know they wanted to meet with us. For many of you this would raise the issue of confidentiality as it did for us. However the employees were so willing to forego confidentiality that they lined up to see us. As a matter of fact there were times when I personally walked out on the floor, where there may be as many as 200 women on sewing machines, and one would stand up, publicly and say "Sarah, have you talked to the counselor about that old man of yours coming in drunk again?" So there was little or no confidentiality among these people.

One of the things, to my knowledge, that we did differently than any other EAP was giving learning disability evaluations when we had a referral for alcohol or drug issues.

One case stands out in my mind more than any other. There was a woman whose name was Edna Mariah (anonymous), most southern women had two names and went by both, was referred to us for production problems. In the course of my interview with her I asked her "what was going on?" She stated that "when we first come here we get paid minimum wage, but we get paid on the basis of piece work as time goes on. I had worked myself up from a minimum wage job of about $5.00 an hour making $200.00 a week. I was very glad to get that job because there were not many in the community."

As an aside, there were a number of school buildings that had been closed as a result of integration and they were available on a lease basis. So Gene

Gwaltney went in and opened up his sewing machine operations in these buildings, and the community had a new source of income.

Getting back to Edna Mariah, she said "gradually I worked myself up to about $15.00 an hour and that was real good money. Since I was a teenager I had been fond of drinking beer, we made a home brew, and so I always had a good supply of beer. I got to the point after a while that I got nervous during the day if I didn't have some beer to drink so I found myself slipping off out to the truck and drinking a little beer. Then one day the supervisor told me I couldn't do that. So I went to see the doctor and the doctor gave me one of them things you call a vallum. That helped a lot, but the problem was, and this is where I got in trouble on the production line, where I was making $15.00 an hour based on production, I went back to the $5.00 an hour. I sewed every one of those pieces, whether it was a shirt or underspants. I sewed 'em all the same. The woman at the end inspecting them said that wasn't acceptable. That's why their sending me to the program."

It was pretty obvious that she had a serious problem with the benzos and the alcohol. We did an evaluation on her which included a learning disability test. We found that she was severely dyslexic. I remember giving her a report and telling her that she had this condition that would interfere with her ability to think and perform. She said, "yeah I know, all my life I been called dummy, cause I can't read like other people and I don't understand like regular folk." I said "no, Edna Mariah that's not true. There's nothing wrong with your thinking, there's nothing wrong with your brain, as a matter of fact it indicates that you are a very bright woman. You have a problem with being able to mentally see written things the same way as other people do and we can teach you how to deal with that." She started to cry and said "are you telling me after all these years I am not a dummy. Yes ma'am, I'm telling you, you are not a dummy."

Now as a follow up on this, she had three little girls. We did the same evaluation on those three children to see if this was a genetic situation which we know sometimes learning disabilities are. One out of the three also had dyslexia. I would like to think that what we did as a result of that service was to stop this young child from going through the same kind of "you're a dummy" attitude that her mother had experienced.

I cite this story because we had psychologists on our staff that actually were capable of doing learning disability testing as we still do today.

In order for you to understand the culture of Alabama at that time, realizing this was pre-integration days, I will cite another incident which took place in Gene Gwaltney's office. He called in some of the companies bus drivers and said to them "look I've been reviewing the welfare rolls of Tallapoosa County and it's outrageous, we have to do something to get these people to work. I want you all to take the busses and drive every back road in the county and when you see adults sitting on the porch you tell them Russell Corporation is hiring people and you are gon'na get paid for doing a good job. We will do the training and will bring you back and forth on the busses."

About a month later I was in the office again and Gene called these same people in and asked "how is our training program going?" "Mr. Gene when they see us coming they run and hide." Gene said "what did you expect, these are second, third, and fourth generation welfare people and they don't even know what working is like. They don't know the benefits and value of self- esteem that goes with that as well as the economics, so what did you expect? Have we got any that have come in?" One of the drivers said "we got two Mr. Gene," to which Gene replied "that's two more off the welfare rolls than we had before, keep the busses running."

Another incident I cite was when George Wallace was standing in the administrative office at the University of Alabama saying that there would never be a Negro that would ever register at the University. Gene Gwaltney's company being the dominant force in Alexander City, Alabama, already had an integrated school system. The reason for this is that he believed as did the Russell's themselves in a strong education system for all the people, regardless of color.

Nancy Gwaltney tells me, in my conversations with her, that she could have attended any school in the United States, but her parents wanted her to go to the mill school like all of the other kids, because they wanted her to understand and be part of that community.

One afternoon Gene called me and said "I want you to find me some remedial reading teachers for the school system." I said, "Gene that's not in our contract. I didn't say this is not my job, but it's not in my contract." This is a good place to illustrate how I learned to meet the client's needs based on Gene Gwaltney's attitude toward change. He was never satisfied with "not my job". He said "I know it's not in your contract, but I want you to find me some remedial reading teachers. There's a problem in my junior high school and if we let it go any further, my kids are going to be graduating, and they're not going to be qualified to work in the mill."

One of the tests they used to determine if a person was eligible for hiring was they gave him a checkbook and said balance this checkbook and then they gave him a newspaper and said read any article and tell me what it said. They wanted their workers to have comprehension and basic mathematical understanding to be able to work in the mills. This worked very successfully.

Going back to the question of the remedial reading teachers, I said "so what happened?" He said "I found out that one of the teachers in our school system doesn't have the best use of the English language and I don't want my employees talking like she does, so go find me at least two or three good remedial reading teachers that we can hire and put on the books".

Another innovative example we did with the Russell account came about because Gene was serving on the Board of Regents for Georgia Tech. One day he called me and Dick Dixon, senior vice president of human resources, into his office and said "I have made arrangements for you and Don to go to Atlanta and do a two day presentation to the Georgia Tech MBA students on Employee Assistance Programs. Dick I want you to talk about the value of it and the benefit we get as far as the company is concerned, and Don I want you to explain what the EAP is and how it works." We did that for several years and as I mentioned previously I discussed this same concept with my classes at LSU.

We had a high rate of recovery for the people who were put into treatment for alcoholism because of the support of the company itself as well as the Gwaltneys and Russells. One of the things that was unique was that there was a house on the grounds that use to be an old executive home but had gone into disrepair. Nancy Gwaltney decided she was going to restore that house and name it the Pelham House. The house was made available during regular working hours for any person in recovery or anyone just wanting information about alcohol or substance abuse. In addition the company also allowed employees to go to AA meetings on the company site during their work hours. Years later we had a number of companies which allowed AA meetings to be held on company premises. Again this was an innovation that came out of the Russell Corporation's EAP services.

Sadly, EAP's no longer have a relationship with senior management. I recognize that time constraints on the workforce precludes a 7 hour training program. However, if senior management is aware, or involved with the EAP, you should have ongoing educational programs on the value of the EAP through the human resources department.

There are many other companies that saw the value of what we did, but saw other issues that needed to be addressed not in the typical EAP. For example, the Louisiana Workman's Compensation Corporation (LWCC) started having serious problems with traumatic injuries in the workplace and then post-traumatic stress claims after that. They called us and asked what we could do to help them. We developed what was one of the first Critical Incident Stress Debriefing (CISD) services in the United States. We traveled all over the country where there had been fatal and/or very serious injuries in the workplace. This service demonstrated very effectively that if the CISD was done properly and then was followed up with post- traumatic stress services that they reduced or eliminated the number of workman's compensation claims.

One of the most interesting and challenging non-EAP services that we were asked to provide was for the Bayou Steel Corporation, which is a major steel mill in Louisiana. This is a union organization. Union and management had reached an impasse and could not agree on the terms of a new contract and therefore there was a lockout on the part of management until the union came to some terms. That strike or lockout lasted about four years. During that time other people were brought in, crossing picket lines, to operate the mill. While the union members were locked out they were not paid wages and not eligible for any benefits.

I discussed this with my staff and then talked to the company and told them our intent to continue to provide services to the union membership. They replied "as long as it's not an official benefit we have no position". We then discussed it with the union officials and told them "even though we were not to be paid for the services during the strike period those services were still available to their people." I made periodic visits to the union hall to remind them this program was still available to them. They used our services to a greater degree during this time then they did under normal circumstances.

When it came time to put this work force back together again, just imagine four years of bitter hostility of crossing the picket line, of people being threatened, and in some cases, fights breaking out among families in the community at grocery stores and other businesses. This was a very hostile environment. You couple that with bringing people back to work in a highly dangerous environment where any tip of an overhead ladle with molten metal could kill or maim a half dozen people.

We were asked to be competitive and put together a bid on how we would approach this. It was interesting that two academic institutions gave some very sophisticated approaches that they would use, but because of our relationship with management and particularly the Union, we were selected to address this. I cited earlier in the EAP's history the unions suspicion of EAP's as a management tool to bypass the grievance process.

The regional vice president of United Steel Workers, Francis Melancon, understood the true value of our EAP. His endorsement of our managing the company drug testing program made it possible for us to have contracts with the steel workers. Francis was my most enthusiastic EAP salesman.

I digress here to share with you some tidbits about Francis. I received a call from him one night around 10:00 p.m. My first reaction was there had been a crisis involving the union. However, it turned out to be a delightful and funny phone call. You have to understand that Francis' last name, Melancon, identified him as a Cajun. I always kidded him about his Cajun accent. The phone call was to let me know he was in Boston going to a union management program at Harvard. My comment was "Oh my God, I'm going to have a Cajun accent mixed with a Harvard enunciation."

Francis was one of the most astute and hardnosed negotiators I ever worked with. Because he lapsed into his Cajun accent during negotiations, the lawyers representing the company assumed he was naïve and uneducated. However, Francis used this to create that impression very successfully. I remember one time specifically when he asked me to sit in on a negotiation and at the break I said to Francis "you don't really expect that they will agree to the terms you have presented." He looked at me and with a wry smile said "mai they tink I'm stupid and are taking advantage of me."

Let me return to the story. We worked first with the union to identify any of the concerns they had and try to deal with the issues we knew would be present when they returned to work. Subsequently we did the same thing with the supervisors and managers.

There were two very interesting things that came out of these sessions, first I remember a supervisor asking me "what are we going to do when they come walking in here with T-shirts saying we won?" I said "It's very simple you say "ok you won now let's get back to work", knowing full well that they had not won everything they had expected to get. The second question was "how are we going to come back together again, it's going to be impossible for us to join hands and sing kumbaya?" My comment was "that was not necessary nor was it expected."

What we did do was emphasize that both sides had one common interest and that was to get back to work and get the mill back in operation, so that everyone could have an income again. The morning that we put these people back together again we told them "you don't have to shake hands, you don't have to do anything, but both sides say let's go to work". Surprisingly there was not one incident that involved any conflict between labor and management as a result of these training sessions.

About a year and a half later, because we managed the Kaiser Corporation account for the state of Louisiana, they had a similar situation when they went out on strike. Again we had the same problems with the union as well as company management. It was interesting that the biggest problem with the union employees were those union members that refused to walk the picket line and got a job elsewhere. They were castigated worse than the management people were.

One of the most dramatic services we were called upon to provide was when the Kaiser Corporation had a huge industrial explosion at the plant, in which 37 employees were injured, five seriously and two critical. We had a problem trying to get past all the federal agencies to go in and do our CISD (Critical Incident Stress Debriefing) work. Finally we were able to get through and do what we normally would have done the first few days. In the mean time we secured a list of all the employees that had been hospitalized and we actually made hospital visits with each of those injured.

I remember the first time we walked into the waiting room and there were union officials there and they asked "why were we here"? I replied "that we are here to provide the EAP services to the employees and their families and to help them get through this." They indicated they did not know this was covered. Technically it's not but it needed to be done. So again what we discovered was that if you let the employee know the company cares, and they follow up with services to the employee and family as well, you change the whole dynamic of the relationship with the employee and the company.

In 1984, Blue Cross came to us, as mentioned in another chapter, and asked us to put together a program to help manage their in-patient and out-patient mental health and substance abuse services. The cost was eating them alive and they weren't sure they were getting the services the people needed. As a result of our skills and ability in counselor training and recognition of signs and symptoms of impairment and what constituted good treatment we were able to successfully put this program together.

One of the other issues that I remember very vividly was with the Allied Corporation, a major client of ours here in Louisiana. We had done a number of interventions using their safety and medical personnel to be part of the intervention team. The corporate office heard of this and were fascinated but yet scared of what we were doing. When they asked how it was working, all of their people who were participating, said it worked very well.

As a result of that I was asked to go to one of their mining operations in Green River, Wyoming to train their supervisors in recognizing signs and symptoms of impairment. In order for you to get a picture of this operation, they were mining a product called Trona, which is a soda potash, which is mined 2000' below the ground. This is the only time I have ever conducted counseling sessions 2000' below ground in an office set aside for that purpose.

When we first met with the union, again this was a United Steel Worker's group, it was a very hostile atmosphere because there had been long time chronic issues between union and management. Most of these issues surrounded drug and alcohol in the workforce. We had a joint meeting with labor and management and explained to them what I was trying to do. The union immediately said "this was BS and we are not going to get caught in this trap and you are trying to get rid of our people." I mentioned this to their president, Paul, who was a very tall, gaunt man who looked like he had been in many a barroom fight. We took a break and he was standing next to me and asked "tell me who you really are? Are you DEA, the sheriff's office, a company pimp?" I responded "I told you I carried a membership in the union years ago so I know what union membership is." So he put his arm around me and said "oh you are one of us." No, I replied, "I'm not one of you nor one of them, I'm here to walk straight down the middle and help your people without being biased or favoring the company in any way."

Fast forward and about two weeks after we established the training program, Paul came to me and said "I have a problem. I have a brother who got fired this morning because he came in drunk." "How many times has this happened?" I inquired. "I think about 4 or 5 times" Paul said. "So they have given him a lot of rope and he hasn't taken advantage of it. What do you want me to do?" I asked. He said "I want you to go see Grover, the general manager, and get my brother rehired." "Paul I can't do that, I won't do that, I am not going to overstep the bounds of the discipline of the supervisor, but I will do this, I will talk to Grover and see if he can find a way to make this work without compromising the authority of the supervisor."

When I went to speak to Grover his first reaction was "no, we've given him all of the chances we want and we are going to fire him; that stands." "Well, I said, this is the first time the union has come to us and I think we have a real opportunity to have a break through and get the union's support." As a matter of fact I got Paul and the union to agree that if this guy goes to treatment and he relapses even once, they will not grieve it and accept the fact that you fired him." Grover said, "You did what? If that is true then we will reinstate him subject to his going to treatment and staying clean and sober." That was the beginning of another five or six employees that I'm not sure we would have ever seen but were referred by the union themselves before the problem got too bad.

My point is that we had a totally different relationship with unions than the usual EAP because unions were suspicious of the EAP as being a company tool.

So, we've had extensive services in other areas that are "not my job". The common denominator in all of these is very simple, did it require some sort of counseling or management skills that we had, that we could accommodate these needs, and the answer was "yes".

I cite all of these examples as issues that "are not my job". Yet we felt that when asked, and we had the skills, or we could develop the skills to meet our customer's need, we could provide those services and that's the reason our program was so successful.

By adopting a model of not using the expression "not my job" but rather of trying to find a solution to meet the client's needs, even though it did not typically fall into the framework of an EAP, it was certainly something that if we had the skills and abilities to do, we provided those services.

So the questions for you are, "when something unusual occurs with a client, do you say "that's not my job?"

As a therapist "are you in a rut and in a comfort zone that will not allow you to find new ways to improve the client's outcome or to meet your client's needs?"

When is the last time you went to a continuing education or university program that added to your clinical skills?

Have you ever challenged the lack of definition of behavioral health and its impact on your practice by saying "that's not my job"?

CHAPTER 8

LEGISLATION

Legislation, as it relates to the content of this book, is driven by three sources. The first is medical necessity. The drive by public opinion that there is a need to address a specific medical problem. An example of this would be the need to address mental health issues and secondarily substance abuse. The second is legislation driven by anti-criminal activity. This is driven by the need to address a criminal action or element. An example of this would be the war on drugs and the incarceration of people for the possession or distribution of illicit drugs. The third source driving legislation is the never ending pursuit of new revenue sources primarily through taxation.

Medical Necessity
There is a public perception that mental health is an ongoing critical crisis in American society. Therefore there is a strong need to provide additional services for the mentally ill. This is in line with the need to use pharmaceuticals for the treatment of a mental illness. Most of the early attempts at addressing this issue were clothed under the title Mental Health Parity. The presumption was that mental health included typical mental health conditions plus substance abuse as well. However time has proven that this is not particularly true.

There have been 28 states up until the present time (2017) that have adopted legislation on mental health parity. One of the earliest states to adopt this legislation was Maine. Interestingly enough the presentation of the need for the mental health parity bill was that it wasn't being treated like a physical illness and therefore it was discrimination legislation against mental health.

However, all of the early so called mental health parity bills were all anti-alcoholism and the hypocrisy was they specifically excluded substance abuse. Substance abuse has traditionally been treated as the red headed step child at the family reunion of mental health.

The first attempt at federal legislation on mental health parity was the Wellstone-Domenici Act. This bill, typical of the state issues, attempted to remediate the anti-discrimination against mental health but the authors of the bill refused to accept that substance abuse was also being discriminated against and they in turn eliminated the substance abuse services from the mental health parity bill.

It's interesting to note that the authors of these bills starting with Maine and also with the federal legislation, reportedly all had family members who were questionably substance abusers but the authors wanted them to be treated as mental illness rather than carry the stigma of substance abuse.

Louisiana has made three attempts at mental health parity bills. The first one, which I was involved in personally, was part of the legislative study group that was appointed to recommend a "mental health parity bill". The study group was brought together under the auspices of then chairman of Health and Welfare, Jim Donelon, who subsequently became the Insurance Commissioner for the state of Louisiana. Of the committee appointed to do the mental health parity bill I was the only one of 24 members that represented the substance abuse community. Obviously the intent was to focus the needed services and legislation toward mental health. This is exactly what came out of the recommendations for new legislation. I wrote a minority opinion requesting that substance abuse be included however it was over-ridden and was never included in the legislation.

The business community specifically LABI (Louisiana Association of Business and Industry) and Blue Cross/Blue Shield of Louisiana were opposed to the mandated benefits required in this legislation. I was serving as chairman of LABI's Health Care Council at the time and was asked to appear before Governor Foster to present an oppositional position and request that he veto the bill since it had been approved by the House and the Senate. It was obvious that there was too much pressure brought from the mental health community, specifically from the psychiatric community and the social workers, that we could not reverse this process. The fact that we proved the bill had been terribly written and that it was going to be very expensive to administer a so-called mental health parity bill, which was only for mental health.

In 2007 under the auspices of Senator Ben Nevers there was another attempt to write a mental health parity bill. Again the mental health people took control of this legislation and excluded substance abuse for the last time. I referenced earlier that 28 states had introduced mental health parity. Most of these bills specifically omitted substance abuse.

The most recent attempt at a mental health parity bill was the ACA, Obamacare, which required services for substance abuse as well as mental health. This was legislation with no teeth in it, since it was not designed to offer substance abuse with same benefits as mental health.

Even now there are still attempts by the federal government to write a truly inclusive mental health and substance abuse legislation. However, even though the bill mandates services for both mental health and substance abuse the problem is that there is not adequate funding for the substance abuse and therefore has no authority. This leaves the millions of people who suffer from substance abuse illness very limited or in some cases non- existent resources. With the public outcry over the "heroin/opioid epidemic" the Trump administration has stopped short of declaring this a national emergency (2017). Time will tell if history repeats itself and this is feel good legislation without adequate funding.

So how does this affect your practice? If you are a mental health practitioner it gives you a foothold into being able to guarantee that you can provide services and be reimbursed for those services to the mentally ill.

There is very little to no major identification of the substance abuse in the parity bills and therefore there are few financial resources to be able to provide these services if you are a practitioner primarily in the substance abuse field.

The net effect of the confusion on mental health and substance abuse services and the problem created by the use of the term "behavioral health" is the focus of this book.

Anti-criminal Legislation.

The need for anti-criminal legislation is to address an illicit or illegal problem. In this instance we are talking about the war on drugs. Unfortunately most of these acts of legislation are motivated out of an intent to punish the patient rather than to provide medical services for them. It is easier to provide legislation that says these people are criminals and forget about the fact that they are driven to criminal activity because of the need to provide relief from their medical substance abuse problem.

There is a strong public opinion with an understanding that any person running for political office on law enforcement, i.e. District Attorney, judges, sheriffs, coroners, are going to be "tough on crime". A perfect example of the extreme of this reaction, and lack of recognition of this being a medical problem, is legislation in Louisiana that was passed in 2014 by the Louisiana legislature under the sponsorship of Senator Dan Claitor. The bill had the strong support of the Sheriff's Association, the coroners, the DA, and the drug courts. The bill I am referencing was designed to address the "growing heroin problem". Without going into all the details of previous laws and legislation, and what ultimately happened in the drafting of this legislation, is this: if you were using heroin, or if you were a pusher, you would receive a 99 year sentence without probation or parole. The bill was passed with the understanding that this was to punish, and get the pusher and distributor off the street. However it is common knowledge that the pusher or distributor are never seen on the street. They always have runners, or the users themselves, selling these drugs. So, the bill has never been successful at reaching what the goal was, the pusher. As a result you have an awful lot of people with possession of heroin because they have a heroin problem and are attempting to treat themselves with it. They are being condemned to 99 years of prison.

How did the heroin problem begin? We did not see a major opioid or heroin problem on the street until we had a shutdown of our pharmaceuticals on the part of the pharmacy's, and the district attorney's and sheriff's offices. While the intent of this movement was to identify people that were pharmacy drug shopping and to stop them from getting drugs legally, i.e. OxyContin, Oxycodone, Lortabs, they now drove them into this sub-culture, or this criminal element, to buy the drugs necessary to treat their addiction. In addition the cost of the pharmaceuticals were substantially higher than the purchase of pure heroin, as a matter of fact, the average cost went from $100 by prescription to $10 on the street.

So, back up, how did all of this opioid difficulty come about? When you stop and see what was happening, was that the medical society under the auspices of and encouragement of so-called remediation of the pain problem, was to put the patient on an opioid treatment, i.e. OxyContin, Oxycodone.

As an additional aside in the treatment of this problem, Louisiana had the highest rate of addiction and use of opioids in the treatment of its workman's compensation patients.

I was appointed by LABI to a governor's commission to represent them in a study of the opioid problem in the workman's compensation field. Again, I was the only person, out of a committee of 25 that had an interest or background in substance abuse. The other members of the committee consisted of lobbyists representing PhRMA, tort attorneys representing the injured worker, the Louisiana Pharmacy Association, physicians providing services in pain management clinics, and a medical psychologist. When the subject came up about Louisiana's high use of opioids and the injured worker, the proposed solution was to tweak the formulary on the use of opioids and then the concern would go away.

I raised the question "what could we do to improve the outcome and shorten the period of disability for the injured worker, and reduce costs of the opioids? The response from the other members of the committee was "who let this guy in?" We had done an in-depth study of this problem with a large workman's compensation company. The study revealed the high percentage of patients that subsequently became addicted as a result of the very loose prescription of opioids for the patient. In the course of the study on the workman's compensation problem, it became obvious that we needed to look at what the pain management community was doing. Pain management physicians wrote the mental health and diagnostic criteria for substance abuse for the workman compensation patient. Nowhere in the DSM or ICD-10 will you find anything written, like the pain management physicians wrote, as being descriptive of addiction. If you read their description you will see that it was specifically designed to anticipate that if they addicted a patient by virtue of their prescribing that they would not be held responsible (Iatrogenic).

There is now a national recognition of the heroin problem in the United States. However, the heroin problem is still dwarfed by the alcoholism problem in this country. The heroin issues have received a higher profile and even some candidates for congress and the presidency have talked about their being strong on offering help rather than punishment for these patients.

New Revenue Taxation.
The other issue that motivates legislation is a need for new revenue taxation resources. An example of this concept goes back to the legislation that was

passed concerning the anti-tobacco campaign. Behind all of these good intentions was a need to capture a huge new source of resources from the taxation of tobacco products.

Many of the states when they finally did have settlements from the tobacco industry set that money aside for the treatment of anti-tobacco use. It was paradoxical that the anti-tobacco tax money was turned around and used for less than anti-tobacco legislation and/or treatment.

In addition it was presented as a way to discourage people from trying to use a tobacco product. However, the legislators also knew this would probably not work and that it would continue to be an ongoing source of revenue for their pet projects. It has certainly been true in Louisiana. An ongoing example of the "sin tax" legislation is the gambling regulations and taxation. In Louisiana, gambling is prohibited by statute. A perfect example of semantics is that the gambling legislation is called "gaming".

I asked my U.S. Senator Bill Cassidy when we met and were discussing the possibility of the proposed medical marijuana legislation at a federal level, "as a physician supporting this, if you could not tax this, would you still have the same interest you profess at the present time?" He looked at me a little quizzically and he said "that could make a difference. However we do know that marijuana has medicinal value in treating certain conditions." I asked him to give me specifics on this and let me know if there were not already pharmaceuticals on the market, i.e. anti-nauseous or glaucoma medication, that were as good as or better than marijuana, and he did acknowledge that there were.

Louisiana recently passed a medical marijuana bill. It's interesting that as conservative a legislature as Louisiana has, this bill would never have passed if it was a stand-alone marijuana bill. So how do you get legislation like this passed? You change the description and intent that is more acceptable from a public policy point of view. Example, if you call this a marijuana bill that was available to people that have medical problems but did not title it medical marijuana, that bill would never have passed. If we go back to the idea of the power of words which we spoke about earlier, in this case, you take a subject that is controversial, i.e. like in the description of Noah Sweats position on alcohol, there's always going to be some opinion about it and that's true of marijuana. How do you get that public perception changed? You dress it up in a new title and have a need, socially or medically, to have the legislation, i.e. medical marijuana.

There is also a strong legislative intent as evidenced by the passage of recreational marijuana in the states of Washington, Oregon, Colorado, Arizona, Alaska, the District of Columbia, and California will soon be added to the list (January, 2018). This bill would never have been passed had it not been dressed-up in the title of "recreational" marijuana. The generally accepted definition of the word "recreation" is that it is fun, that it is legal, has public acceptance, and is consequence free. The proponents of recreational marijuana legislation have introduced another definition which states "relating to or denoting drugs taken on an occasional basis when socializing."

So how did we find ourselves in a situation where the legality of marijuana has become a prominent issue in the legislature and public opinion? Does public attitude and legislation create an addiction problem of tsunami proportions in this country?

You have to go back to the time when marijuana was generally illicit and you kind of looked the other way, in the so-called hippie generation. These are people who are now in their fifties, sixties, or older who did not stop using marijuana as they aged. The poster child for this phenomenon is Willie Nelson. This became an example to the millennial generation that said that "if they can use it and it's not so bad we can too." My own patients, especially my millennials (15, 18, 20 year olds), when I ask them about marijuana, what they know about it, they tell me that they know more about it than I do. They tell me that it is no worse than alcohol.

When I try to explain to them the effect marijuana has on the brain, they don't want to listen. Their position is that it's not as bad as alcohol and it doesn't really do anything to the brain except "mellow me out". They are not willing to accept that marijuana is a sedative drug, and that it has initial and long term effects on the cognitive skills of the marijuana user. Example, when I ask them "what is glutamate?" they look at me quizzically and ask if this is a test? My response is that glutamate is a natural drug created by the brain to help you learn new things and to prompt your memory. When you use marijuana you have effectively blocked the successful use of glutamate. What you have done is shut down the ability to recognize and learn new things and you certainly have a block as far as memory is concerned about the negative consequence of the use of marijuana.

There has been an attempt to re-write the diagnostic criteria for marijuana by saying that since you don't experience a physical withdrawal you can't truly have an addiction. For those people who make that comment, I wish they would sit in my office and see the effect that long term and early use of marijuana, starting at 14 or 15 years of age, and continuous use of it, has had on the brain scholastically, their employment potential, or the diminishing of their ambition and functioning in life experiences.

So do we see the use of legislation to change public opinion, to create new opportunities for taxation, and hopefully new opportunities for treatment of people that are suffering from mental health and addiction? The extent that this legislation resolves itself positively will determine the successful outcomes of treatment for mental health and substance abuse. There are numerous references to the term "behavioral health" in legislation but nowhere is it defined clinically.

So what does the term "behavioral health" mean?

Does this legislation change your attitude on addiction?

Does this legislation improve the outcome for your patients?

Does it increase your income?

CHAPTER 9

FEEDING THE DRAGON

Folklore and mythology and currently science fiction tells us of the existence of great flying creatures called dragons. There were two types of dragons, one that was good and had been tamed by man and was used to protect against the second, which was the bad dragon that was attempting to devour them. However both dragons shared one thing in common, they had a terrible insatiable appetite that had to be constantly fed.

Whether we believe in dragons or not it is a good vehicle to demonstrate the development of health insurance and the problems associated with the development and improvement of health care services. The analogy of the dragon and health care is a parallel story between great benefits derived from the taming of the dragons to be used against the bad dragons that consumed insurance dollars, but at what cost, because of the appetite that had to be constantly fed.

According to an Open Minds article behavioral health spending reached $213.6 billion last year-for an increase of $25.2 billion or 13.4% since 2011. The majority of that total was for mental health services, which accounted for 84% or $195.6 billion in spending.

In order to understand how health care services have developed we need to go back to see how payment of the delivery system, and by whom, the services were provided.

Prior to the time of the Greeks and Romans we begin to have some fairly sophisticated systems of understanding of both physical and mental health issues.

There was strong evidence in earlier societies that there were people who were considered experts or considered to be helpful in providing health services. They were referred to as a Shaman, witch doctor, medicine man or woman, or simply a healer. (As an aside, a patient of mine told me I was a shaman. I asked what he meant by that and his response was "you bring people through dark and scary places back into the light." I have always thought this was one of the greatest titles by which I could be called.) Surprisingly these early people had a good understanding of basic physical anatomy, broken bones, and injured muscles, but they also had a detail understanding of the use of plants and minerals to provide health services. As an example, it is commonly known that they used willow leaves and willow bark to make a tea used for pain medication. They also used cherry bark to help with coughs and colds. Flowers like marigolds were used to provide relief from minor burns, eczema and bruising. These early health care providers spoke in terms of spirits. Spirits meaning those parts of the body or those things that had invaded the body that affected the physical and/or the mental health of the person. From the very beginning we have an understanding that there was two separate and distinct issues that needed to be treated, the physical ailments as well as the mental ailments.

If we fast forward from the earlier history of health care to what we consider today to be modern health care, my earliest recollections were during the depression. I lived in the country and as a result we did not see many old Model T Fords because few people had an automobile. Doctors made house calls either on horseback or in buggies. When it came time to pay for services, the doctor left the house with a buckboard of salted or smoked hams, a couple of chickens hanging from the saddle, or some eggs or vegetables from the garden. Much of this early reimbursement for health services was done on a barter basis.

The precursor to modern health insurance began with "mutual aid societies" in the 1870's. In 1929 the first true health insurance plan (Blue Cross Plans) was developed in Texas as a joint venture between hospitals and the Texas State Teachers Association. In 1930 Blue Shield was formed to cover the costs of surgeons. In 1935, the National Labor Relations Act was the catalyst for employer based health insurance as it was now seen as an effective and valuable benefit to workers. Blue Cross and Blue Shield companies began to empower more working Americans to access the healthcare system. In 1939, the first true employer based health insurance plans was designed by The Equitable Life Assurance Society. World War II proliferated the growth of health insurance as an acceptable benefit to labor in lieu of salary freezes.

I spoke earlier about the question of the appetite of the dragon and the appetite of the health care system. The following two examples are cited to demonstrate what's happening in health care.

I ran across a copy of the nursery charges for my wife when she was born in 1930. The charges read "service for 1 normal female infant per day of nursery – charge 50 cents. I recently checked with two of our larger health insurance plans on what the same charge would be today for a normal healthy baby. The prices ranged from $1500.00 to $1800.00 per day. This is not to say however that the services available if need be were not more sophisticated and better than 1930. A second example are the charges for a routine appendectomy. In 1933 the charges were $143.75 which included a $50.00 surgical fee and a $2.00 electric fan fee for the operating room. Today, one hospital reported on the low end of $7500.00 for an appendectomy which included $1600.00 for the surgeon's charges.

Does this mean we should go back to the "good old days" prior to the day of modern medicine or prior to the day of modern conveniences. Who would want to go back to the "good old days" when there was no electricity and you read by lamplight or warmed your house by use of a fireplace, or you did not have running water, or internal plumbing. I know no one who would want to go back to those days. Nor would we want to go to the days when we had to walk or ride a horse or buggy because there were few automobiles.

In today's society when you talk to young people and try to describe what life was like back in the 20's, 30's, and 40's, they look at you as if you are making those stories up. It's hard, if not impossible, for them to visualize that there was no TV, radio, automobiles, or any modern electronic conveniences we know today. Life expectancy in 1930 was age 63 for women and age 59 for men. Those numbers today reflect a life expectancy for women of 82.8 and 79 for the male counterpart.

More than just the life expectancy extension, the quality of life has greatly improved as a result of modern medicine and medications. There have been tremendous strides and improvements in surgical techniques, in diagnostic techniques with radiology, and other technological advances, as well as new medications that have been effective in dealing with some of the physical medical problems. Not so necessarily in the mental health piece which we will describe in detail later.

There is a perception, and attitude, on the part of the public and medical community that differentiates between physical medicine and mental health substance abuse medicine. The perception is that the mental health and the substance abuse is more self- induced as opposed to the physical medicine problem. Yet when we look at what the pharmaceutical costs are at the present time, the mental health pharmaceuticals are second only to the top medical problem prescribed. Is this giving you a better outcome on your patients as a result of the use of a medication approach rather than a cognitive or counseling approach?

In my seminars on mental health and substance abuse, I ask this question at the very beginning and I will ask it of you now. How many of you believe that we have a serious alcohol or drug problem in the United States? In the programs that I present, the audience without exception, when I preference how many in the United States, almost every hand goes up and believes there is a serious problem. When I bring it down to Louisiana, those same number of hands are raised. When I come to Baton Rouge, the same number of hands go up but maybe not quite as many. But when I ask if you believe there is a serious problem in your neighborhood with alcohol and drugs, not as many hands go up. The last question is how many of you believe there is a problem with alcohol and drugs in your family or workplace.

Now rarely do we find it but sometimes there are people who are willing to disclose there is a problem in their family or workplace, but most of the time they don't raise their hands. At that point I say let me explain to you what's happened here. We have roughly 320 million people in the United States and I don't know all of those people and neither do you, so yeah they have a problem. In Louisiana we have roughly 4 million people. I don't know all of them either, so yeah they have a problem. Baton Rouge has a population of roughly 230,000 and again I don't have a personal relationship with all these people so yeah they have a problem. The closer I get to where I really live or work, where my own interests and concerns are, the more likely I am to be more sensitive to it.

When we go back and review the number of dollars being spent on alcohol and drugs in the Unites States and the number of people that are suffering from alcohol and drug issues, which SAMHSA indicates is roughly 10%, with another 10% from mental health problems. This means that 20% of the people suffer from some sort of substance abuse or mental health problem.

However, that's not the real number. We know that for every person who has a serious mental illness or substance abuse problem they affect and infect another four people. Those people are spouses, family members, brothers, sisters, children, friends, employers, and the list can go on. Basically for each person who has this illness there are four others specifically affected by it.

Let's go back and do the numbers again. If you have 300 million people in the United States and 20% suffer from these conditions that is 60 million people. If we attribute the other number I gave you, affecting four additional people, now we are talking about four times 60 million, which is 240 million. Now we have roughly ¾ of the population of the United States that is affected or infected by every person who has a mental illness or substance abuse problem. As of January 15, 2015, the gross spending for pharmaceuticals was $373.9 billion. Lost wages and economic costs to businesses from mental health is staggering. A wakeup call for the public and in particularly business are the statistics on depression. It is reported that one in four women in the workforce report being depressed and 82% of the workforce reported depression affected their productivity. Antidepressants are the most common prescription medication for Americans age 18-44, and the third most common drug across all ages. So, what do these numbers mean, apparently not enough to take action.

SAMHSA reports that by the year 2020, mental and substance abuse disorders will surpass all physical diseases as a major cause of disability worldwide. Here are some additional statistics which should serve as a wakeup call to you as a therapist. U.S. spending on medicines is forecast to reach $610-$640 billion by 2020. U.S. health care spending grew 5.8% in 2015, reaching $3.2 trillion or *$9,990 per person.*

How do these numbers impact the business sector? Depression is a major cause of disability, absenteeism, presenteeism, and productivity loss among working age adults. 70% of health care costs can be attributed to the decline of productivity due to absenteeism and presenteeism. Depression alone is estimated to cost $83 billion annually in the United States and in terms of presenteeism, the disorder is the highest cost health condition nationwide. Presenteeism is a term used by human resources to describe the lack of performance by the employee due to physical, mental, and personal problems. The cost of depression to employers in lost work days is as great or greater than the cost of many other medical conditions, including heart disease, diabetes, or back problems.

What does this mean to you as a therapist? Two thoughts I have, are first, strong clinical need for your services and secondly, does the term "behavioral health" help to identify the specifics of the public attitude to the spending problem. If action, means anything, the term "behavioral health" has not helped in solving the problem because it has blurred the lines between physical medicine and mental health.

I don't know about you but the numbers I gave about the cost due to loss of wages, loss of income, costs of pharmaceuticals, and hospitalization for these two elements don't fit in my checkbook. What point am I trying to make –as long as we focus on the numbers, the statistics, instead of the faces; until we can translate all of those numbers into faces where the person that we see is really truly a person in our life, then that begins to make sense and we find the most effective way to present this, in a clinical way, is to help people recognize signs and symptoms of what is going on. Once we have established that there is a face instead of a number, we are more likely to change our attitude on how to deal with this problem.

This is also true of the attitude towards and recognition of our patient that has a substance abuse condition.

So has this chapter helped you understand a little better how health insurance works? Will it help you to have a better outcome with your patient and your income?

Remember the story that I started with about the dragons, the dragons serve a great purpose, particularly the good dragons that protected mankind, but the bad dragons had this terrible appetite as well. So, the appetite we are feeding with respect to the cost of our gross national product is going to consume us if something is not done. Doing something doesn't mean that we stop providing these services or providing medications that are necessary. What is does mean is that we get a better result if we use better treatment modalities than the ones we are currently using. Until that happens the costs of services are going to continue to escalate. Currently, health care services makeup 17.8% of the GDP. Again let me reiterate what SAMHSA reported "that by the year 2020, mental and substance use disorders will surpass all physical diseases as a major cause of disability worldwide".

Does the term "behavioral health" describe what SAMHSA is reporting in this announcement?

How does the term "behavioral health" explain how this change will occur?

The pharmaceutical industry will continue to promote the idea of behavioral health because it allows them to advertise every condition is best treated by a pill. As long as physicians, insurance companies, employers, and individuals accept or believe there is a magic bullet for every condition, the problem will escalate. So we need to identify "What the Hell is Behavioral Health?

CHAPTER 10

FACTORS INFLUENCING DIAGNOSIS/REIMBURSEMENT

This chapter begins the conflict and questions of "What the Hell is Behavioral Health?" In addition it also reviews the validity of the term dual-diagnosis. An understanding of this evolution of "behavioral health" will set the tone for treatment of your patient/client and subsequent reimbursement.

In 1980 Blue Cross came to Hidalgo Health Associates for help on managing in-patient services for mental health and substance abuse issues. They came to us for our skill and experience with providing EAP services for their own employees. I spent six months reviewing the entire system from the time the phone rings stating the provider wanted to admit a patient for services until the patient's discharge. The Blue Cross nurse was not equipped to deal with these problems, i.e. patient is suicidal, pass go, collect your $200.

We developed a whole system for review starting with diagnosis, severity of problem, appropriate level of service, continued stays, and discharge.

One of the complaints against review companies was that non-physicians were making clinical decisions. All of our final decisions were made by psychiatrists.

Early in this process, there were some 20 providers complaining about the per diem reimbursement rates and the treatment of outlier cases. A meeting was called to address these issues and I was asked to participate. During introductory remarks I was not identified as to why I was in attendance. The providers' complaint was that reimbursement rates were based on studies done by Blue Cross and therefore were biased in favor of the lower reimbursement rates. The lead actuary for the providers stated that their independent studies showed a wide disparity between the Blue Cross rates and what the reimbursement should be. I asked him "Who did the report?", and he said "CADA." When I asked him if this was the report he was referencing— I just happen to have a copy in my briefcase— he said "yes that's exactly the report that we're talking about that supports our position of additional reimbursement." I asked if he had read the summary of this report. He said "what do you mean?" My reply was "let me quote it to you, it says there is no appreciable difference in the successful outcome between a 30 day in-patient treatment program and an out-patient program. So why should Blue Cross pay you a higher per diem for an in-patient program than for an out-patient program?" He then said, "No, that was not the correct study that had been done" and yet he had quoted exactly from the study that I had given to him. After a few more hours of discussion it was clear that we were at a loggerhead and were not going to resolve this problem.

Joe Manry, senior vice president of Blue Cross Provider Reimbursement, asked for a break in the meeting and asked me to go outside and talk with him. He said, "Don if we take out the outliers, which was the main bone of contention off the table for this provider group, can you protect us from the long term stays. I looked at him and said Joe, do you have that much confidence in our staffs ability to be able to provide an adequate yet reasonable documentation of length of stay for you. He commented, if you tell me you can do it, I believe it. I said Joe the only way that I'll do this is if you let me write and include a hold harmless clause to go into every contract that you have with every provider that's in that room. He said, what do you mean? I told him I had to have a hammer that I hold them to a certain level of acceptance and that level will be what I draft as hold harmless." To my knowledge I was the one to put together the first hold harmless clause included in those contracts.

Basically the hold harmless clause said that unless we, the utilization review company, could approve the admission and/or stay of a patient they would not be reimbursed. Further the provider could not sue the patient, Blue Cross, or us for their charges, and in effect it was a hold harmless in all phases. We resumed the meeting and Joe said let's see what we can do about the outlier problem on the table and then he threw out the idea of hold harmless. They jumped on that once they heard there would be a waiver on the outlier fees. All they could think of is now we have a guarantee we can go the longer terms. It wasn't until about two weeks later that they realized what they had signed and then wanted to go to court and challenge the hold harmless clause. The courts did a summary judgement and threw the challenges out. This was the primary way we were able to control and work with the providers from that point on.

In spite of the obvious disagreements and conflict of interest, we worked out a very amicable arrangement between our utilization review physicians and nurses, and the provider treatment programs. We did this by giving them copies of our manual, saying this is what we will be following. In addition we did seminars for all of their staff so we were all on the same page. Obviously this did not resolve all of the problems but it did cut down on the number of appeals filed.

We overcame the concern by the providers that a non-physician was making the medical diagnosis and recommendations for their patients. Our system was worked on the following basis: our psych nurses were trained in how to use this manual and they had the authority to approve a case, but could not disapprove it. If there was a question about the appropriateness of stay or length of stay or diagnosis this must be turned over to a psychiatrist with a copy of all the patients' medical records. At one point we had eleven psychiatrists, all prominent in Louisiana, that were working with us on an individual basis, as consultants, to review these cases.

As further evidence to guarantee that we made every effort to provide the right information, once a year, on a Saturday, from 9 a.m. until 4 p.m. we brought our entire staff, psychiatrists, nurses, and administrative personnel together for an in-service. Each psychiatrist was to give us a short 15 minute presentation on a specific area that needed up dating or creating a new diagnostic criteria and/or length of stay criteria. We documented that we were on task of keeping current on all of the innovative ideas being presented.

The Utilization Review service covered all of the PPO and HMO networks that Blue Cross had, which was approximately 500,000 lives, and as a result of the success with Blue Cross basic services we were awarded the federal employee programs for whom Blue Cross had responsibility. This was an additional 100,000 people. So at one point we probably had between 600,000 and 700,000 lives that we were responsible for to provide utilization review.

Initially all admissions were either mental health or substance abuse. Seldom, and I would be hard pressed to recall any over the first ten years we were doing utilization review work, were there any questions, or use, of the terms "dual diagnosis" or "co-morbid" conditions. Everything was mental health or substance abuse. These two terms have now morphed into "behavioral health." So how has this change affected your practice? I suggest it does not meet the mental health or substance abuse patient's needs.

We kept very accurate records on the documentation of the number of true substance abuse cases, true psychiatric cases. As previously mentioned we did not see or hear the expression of dual diagnosis or co-morbid conditions until after the passage of the mental health parity bills.

Mental health parity bills as previously described, and Louisiana statutes were the same that you had to cover the mental health part of the health insurance plan as any other illness, but it specifically excluded substance abuse. Therefore we no longer had a mandate that had to cover substance abuse as well as mental health.

Here was the dilemma that the treatment people found themselves in. If you were the hospital administrator or the psychiatrist in charge of the treatment and were faced with giving a primary diagnosis of a mental health condition, i.e. major depression, or a diagnosis of substance abuse (alcoholism), one gave you 45 days of in-patient service the other gave you zero. This is not a condemnation of the providers however it does indicate there was a strong economic drive to make sure they had a psychiatric diagnosis along with a substance abuse.

Gradually since the early 2000's we begin to see a proliferation of the terms "dual diagnosis or co-morbid" conditions.

One of the things that happened in this was that we no longer saw any true treatment for the substance abuse patient since all the emphasis in documentation and charting had to indicate that it supported the idea of a psychiatric diagnosis, otherwise the claim would be questioned or denied.

The best example I can give you is a case I personally handled even though I had decreased my involvement since the early days of utilization review. I got a phone call from a treatment center because I was responsible for the company's position, in which they were questioning a diagnosis. I spoke with their psychiatrist, looked at the files, and determined this was a true substance abuse case, the substance being cocaine. The doctor working the case insisted the diagnosis should be major depression. It had nothing to do with cocaine. I reviewed the file and pointed out to him the patient had an ulcerated septum as a result of snorting cocaine, and a fistula that is about to penetrate the brain, and yet you say this is not cocaine. He replied "No, this is strictly major depression." I had to explain to him that the company who bought this policy had a specific prohibition against coverage of substance abuse. My comment was very straight forward, "doctor, your patient needs services, but I cannot violate the contract and what the company is paying for." He still insisted this was not a substance abuse case.

Let me digress for a second. When I was young my grandfather used to treat me like I was an adult. I remember one of the conversations I had with him and he said "son, some day you will be old enough to make your own decisions, and people will test you and your judgement, as to whether or not you know the difference between someone peeing in your ear or if it is raining." That's the way he put it to me. So I told this doctor after some discussion that I needed to share with him what my grandfather had told me. He said "if someone would pee in my ear and told me it was raining, I had to have sense enough to know if it was raining", and doctor "it ain't raining". He reported me to the Louisiana Psychiatric Association for unprofessional conduct. I cite this case simply because it was so flagrant and so much a problem of substance abuse not mental health issues that had been created by the disparity within the mental health parity bills.

As was previously cited, up until the year 2000 we saw little or no questions about dual diagnosis, after that we began to see more and more "dual diagnosis". Today if you ask a treatment center "what is the ratio of your dual diagnosis compared with your straight alcohol or mental health problems?" The response will be somewhere between 60% and 80% of our patients are dual diagnosis.

As further evidence of how we can go from 0 to 60% to 80% dual diagnosis, I cite the following. We were asked to provide an audit on about 1000 patient charts (not our own) that were being administered by another insurance company. There was a bias in favor of the mental health diagnosis for whatever reason. Two of my licensed counselors and myself reviewed about 1000 charts. There was an absolute instruction, at the very beginning, that you will not comment on any substance abuse or alcohol issues if you find them in this report. They will be reported as a mental health problem or dual diagnosis.

If you decide in the very beginning what the diagnosis is and ignore what the facts are, you will wind up with the 60% to 80% dual diagnosis. Our studies from the years, 1980 until 2006, based on over 17,000 reviews of lives, indicated you may have as much as 20% to 25% of all so-called dual diagnosis, are true dual diagnosis.

This would not be bad if we were getting better results from either the psychiatric admissions or the substance abuse admissions. Unfortunately it did not give us a better outcome of either condition. Prior to the time we are talking about, the ratio of successful treatment for substance abuse, this is back in the 1950's through the 1980's is that approximately 50% of the people who went through a substance abuse treatment program would wind up in recovery, the other 50% would relapse and perhaps comeback later on. Today, those same treatment centers, and we document all of this in our own EAP services, will run less than 25%, perhaps as low as 10%, of the people who go through treatment will stay abstinent from drugs and/or alcohol. I recently spoke with Dr. Jon Grant, JD, MD, MPH, who presented at a local conference I was attending and asked him about the success ratio of treatment. His experience is extensive in treatment research and outcomes. He affirmed the 10% success rate of patients in today's treatment centers.

It is my firm conviction based on these studies that we have destroyed the focus on the true nature of the problem, in most cases, that has a primary diagnosis of alcoholism by contaminating it with a "dual diagnosis" and subsequently the patient gets neither the adequate treatment for the mental health condition or the substance abuse condition.

So I ask you again, "What impact do these numbers have on your practice?" "Do you ask the right questions to determine what the true diagnosis should be?" "Do we have our own biases as to how we want to see that diagnosis?" Perhaps we do, but there is criteria we can use that would be more clinically appropriate if we follow that particular criteria. Again, does the term "behavioral health" address the issues of mental health versus substance abuse and does this produce a better outcome? Is your patient and your practice being better served by an accurate diagnostic criteria and a treatment that is appropriate to that patient's condition? Does the dual diagnosis approach give you a better outcome?

Among other balances to find equilibrium in behavioral health treatment is that we have to consider the impact of the DRG's. Diagnostic Related

Grouping's was a method that changed reimbursement for hospitals from a provider directed stay to a diagnostic group definition stay. Prior to this approach the physician would determine how long the patient needed to be hospitalized. Example: patient is admitted for an appendectomy and the doctor decides the hospital stay is 6 days. The DRG formula prescribed 4 days of hospitalization. The DRG's concept came about because of Yale University studies on illnesses and surgeries requiring hospitalization to determine the optimum hospitalization services.

The DRG's could be either a money maker for the providers or a monetary loss. Example: if the patient described in the appendectomy example could be sent home after 1 or 2 days, the hospital would still be reimbursed for the full 4 days; if on the other hand, the hospital kept the patient for more than 4 days, those days were at the hospital's expense.

I contacted Yale to determine if they had in fact considered the DRG formula for mental health and substance abuse stays. They told me they had looked at it but it could not be quantified in the same way as "hot appendix". They told me that someone from Massachusetts General Hospital had interest in the formula. The name of the physician given me was not the one I was connected to when I called the hospital, however it was the right one for the information I was seeking. Dr. David Gastfriend, psychiatrist and director of the Addiction Research Program answered the phone himself. I explained what I was looking for and he told me to contact the Cleveland Health Plan since they had developed the first set of medical necessity criteria in substance use disorders. I did as he suggested, got the answers I needed, and established a relationship with Dr. Gastfriend. In fact, he became the first medical director of our utilization review services.

So as we review the history, attitude, and treatment for mental health and substance abuse from 1980 to the present, do we get a better outcome as a result of the use of dual diagnosis or co-morbid and how does this fit into the definition of behavioral health?

CHAPTER 11

PHARMACEUTICALS (A GAME CHANGER)

One, two, three, four, five, six, seven. I think that's a new record for commercials in between breaks on TV. There were four commercials for a pharmaceutical product in a row. The pharmaceutical industry has changed the way physicians have practiced in the United States.

This book would not have been written, or certainly no emphasis placed on pharmaceuticals, if I had not attended a conference at Arizona State University in Phoenix. The conference was directed primarily at psychologists with focus on how mental health, particularly how psychologists were being manipulated by the pharmaceutical industry, and by use of the term "behavioral health".

This conference was the brain child of Dr. Nicholas Cummings. Dr. Cummings has the reputation for being an innovator in the behavioral health field. He was founder of American Biodyne, a major player in the EAP field, and served as president of the American Psychological Association. He was the chief psychologist for Kaiser/Permanente Health Plan of Northern California (a large HMO). Cummings was hired by Sidney Garfield, the Kaiser Permanente medical director at the time, because Garfield believed "psychiatrists were ultimately physicians and would fall back on being physicians rather than psychotherapists who would understand and treat somatizing patients psychologically instead of medically." (Cummings, 2013, p. 64)

This work was extended by Dr. Michael Hoyt, a prominent psychologist who worked for 35 years at Kaiser Permanente in Northern California. I met

Dr. Hoyt a number of years ago at a seminar he presented in Houston, Texas. I had six of my staff with me at the conference. Dr. Hoyt showed us that it was possible to involve the patient/client in therapy even before they had their first appointment, and described a brief therapy model with clear goals and methods that could make most counseling effective within the 1-10 range typical for EAP work. He has published many books on the topic (e.g., Hoyt, 1995, 2000), and a collection of Dr. Hoyt's papers, Brief Therapy and Beyond: Stories, Language, Love, Hope, and Time (2017) has recently been published. Over the years we have developed both a personal and professional relationship.

Returning to the conference in Arizona, the highpoint in my opinion, was the presentation on pharmaceuticals by Robert Whitaker, a Pulitzer Prize medical research writer on pharmaceuticals. His book, *Anatomy of an Epidemic*, should be a wakeup call for every professional in the mental health field and in particular those of us providing EAP services.

His book exposes the impact of pharmaceuticals starting at the age of 3, when children are being prescribed mind-altering drugs. He tracks the impact of these drugs from infancy to geriatrics. I came home both angry and scared of what was happening as a result of the shift from traditional individual counseling to pharmaceutical treatment for the American public.

What is most important is that his research is objective and international in its scope and publications. As an example, he cites *Lancet*, the British equivalent of the *New England Journal of Medicine* on depression. *Lancet* is a weekly peer reviewed general medical journal. There is additional in-depth research publications in France and Italy, which challenged the American accepted use of pharmaceuticals instead of mental health therapy for the treatment of depression. He also cites the University of Texas, Department of Psychiatry, who challenged the American Psychiatric Associations research on the efficacy of the use of pharmaceuticals for depression. He points out that in most studies favoring pharmaceuticals the testing was conducted by research programs sponsored by grants from the pharmaceutical industry. Mr. Whitaker's book, *Anatomy of an Epidemic*, is a must read for every physician, pharmacist, and mental health practitioner.

An example of the acceptance of drugs to treat depression was demonstrated when Diane Sawyer of CBS 60 Minutes interviewed an independent researcher on the efficacy of drugs on depression. When he said that drugs were at best a placebo, Diane Sawyer challenged him by replying that she had a history of depression and used drugs to treat her condition. In response, he pointed out the power of the placebo effect. He then reminded her that there was a caution by the pharmaceuticals not to discontinue this medication without a doctor's approval. In effect, the medication has induced an iatrogenic condition now creating a dependency on the medication. Ms. Sawyer cited a contradictory survey, as it turned out the survey she cited, was paid for by the pharmaceutical industry, as opposed to the three studies questioning the use of drugs for depression by three independent research groups.

So how has the pharmaceutical industry changed the way medication is prescribed? The following is a description of this marketing strategy.

Many years ago you would have had a salesman, referred to as a detail man, call on a physician and say in effect "Doctor my company has perfected this new medication for this particular condition; here are a few samples we would like for you to try on your patients." Medicine years ago was directed more from the physician to be in charge, while today it appears that the pharmaceuticals have taken over. In substituting the pharmaceutical or medication approach to the behavioral or mental health approach has been to great extent the downfall of the mental health and substance abuse practitioners and the EAP's.

How was this accomplished? To begin with the pharmaceuticals capitalized on the concept that there is a magic bullet for every condition. This additionally capitalized on human behavior to believe that there is a softer, easier way to deal with the problem, i.e. don't tell me to change my eating pattern to avoid being obese, don't tell me I have to exercise to reduce my blood pressure, don't tell me I have to stop drinking in the way I have become accustomed to, in other words, in the simplest terms, it's give me the magic pill that will take care of the problem so that I don't have to exert any changes in my life.

The problem with the mental health and substance abuse field is that it has been considered to be a secondary problem in the medical community. We will discuss this in more detail in the chapter on Deep Capture. As a result no importance was given to behavioral changes. The consequences of that failure is pronounced in the notice from SAMHSA which reported that by the year 2020, that mental health and substance abuse disorders will exceed that of physical medicine diseases.

Man has sought the magic elixir or the magic bullet since time immemorial. It was not until the mid-1800's that the principle was finally accepted based on a series of tests, and developing an agent to attack a particular virus, microbe, or bacteria. The principle was to kill the offending bacteria only and leave the rest of the tissues intact without any damage.

When I ask physicians under the age of 65, does the number 606 have any significance? They look at me quizzically and say "is this a trick question?" When I ask that same question of a physician over the age of 65 many of them will give you a sly smile and say yes. They know that the number 606 was the name of the drug that was tested on multiple animals before it was perfected. Ironically enough, the medication that was developed by Dr. Paul Ehrlich was designed to attack a serious social and medical problem at this particular time which cut across all social strata. This medicine was perfected to replace the use of mercury in the treatment of syphilis.

So how far back do we have to go before we begin to realize the impact of the pharmaceutical industry? History tells us, going back to the earliest times of man, that there was always a Shaman, or witch doctor, or medicine man or woman, which was held in high esteem by the different historical societies. They were experts in concocting some sort of a magical elixir and/or a psychological approach to convincing the patient that they had the skills to cure them. These people capitalized on the magic elixir concept.

In our early American history many of these were known as "snake oil salesmen". These were people that traveled with circus caravans or in medical wagons of their own, pronouncing magical elixirs in this little bottle that would cure anything from ingrown toenails to dandruff and everything in between (most of these elixirs had a high alcohol content). In addition there is a copy of an illustration that shows the use of early settlers and their belief in the ability of magic elixirs. You will note that this appears in an 1897 Sears Roebuck catalog (p. 41) advertising that these products "are valuable to have in every household". One of the major items advertised was a bottle of Laudanum. Laudanum, as you may know, was an almost pure opiate concoction. It was sold without any warning of the possibility of addiction, as a matter of fact, addiction was probably not known or was certainly not considered to be a medical problem. The value of the Laudanum was that it relieved pain almost instantaneously.

History also points out that many other famous practitioners, recommended medications that were supposed to be a panacea for certain conditions. For example, Sigmund Fraud recommended that cocaine was the perfect treatment for many of the illnesses or mood problems that people experienced.

Among those patients treated by Dr. Fraud was the great mystery writer, Oliver Wendell Holmes. Unfortunately, the fact that cocaine was a very addictive drug was not known at that time.

In my own personal experience, I have had the opportunity to work with Dr. Joseph Pursch, a Yugoslavian immigrant psychiatrist. Dr. Pursch was the founder of the Navy Alcoholism Program in California. This facility subsequently became the Betty Ford Treatment Program. I remember one episode in which I was present when he was addressing a group of physicians and in his heavy Yugoslavian accent said, "The problem with you psychiatrists is that you think alcoholism is a Valium deficiency."

So who is the father of modern pharmacy? You go back to the year 200 B.C. in which there was a Greek physician, a part of the Hippocratic physicians, by the name of Galen of Pergamon. Galen was considered to be the authority on physical medicine as well as medications, from the year 200 B.C. until 1800 A.D., a period of 2000 years. His influence was so strong that even until today when you see his name written in the lower case (galenic), some pharmacists recognize it immediately as a concoction of herbs, minerals, and plants that Dr. Galen had formulated. He believed that if one medication did good, a combination of two was better, and if two was good, four was better, and if four was good, eight is better, and on and on.

Today we have this same principle being applied with respect to psychiatric medication. For example, you will see commercials that say try this medication and if that doesn't work we will add this medication and if that doesn't work we will add a third medication. So there is always some additional magic bullet that will take care of the problem.

Can we lay all of the blame for the change in the mental health substance abuse practice at the feet of the medical or pharmaceutical industry? The answer to that question is both yes and no. Yes, because they recognize that human behavior being what it is, does not want to change anything. They want the magic bullet.

If we go back to the original premise of this chapter in which we talked about how medicine was practiced many years ago and we look at how medicine is practiced today, it's almost a guarantee that pharmaceuticals are going to be the way physicians practice.

For example, look at the time constraints placed on a physician, the number of patients they expect to see during a days practice is anywhere from 40 to 60 patients. It becomes impossible for them to do the traditional type of practice of medicine by virtue of history and observation. So now when a patient comes in and says "doctor, I am bummed out, I feel depressed, give me something for that, let me have Prozac."

In effect the patient is dictating both the diagnosis and treatment plan, specifically the pharmaceutical that is needed to medicate his condition. He was educated on this by the TV commercials. In fairness to the physician why is this happening? Is it time constraints to be able to deal with this, or is it the unwritten threat that if the physician does not give him the medication asked for, the patient will then seek out another physician.

A major complication in prescribing mental health medications is that much of the medication for mental health conditions are prescribed by physical medicine physicians, not mental health practitioners, i.e. family practitioners, OB-GYN, orthopedics and internists. In many cases, these physicians are poorly trained to identify psychological problems and have little time to devote to dealing with these issues (Psychology Today, 2014).

It should be noted that multiple studies have been done demonstrating the return on investment of the successful use of an EAP to deal with mental health issues. SAMHSA reports the following: a $7,750 savings per employee at Warner Corporation, because of lower recruitment and training costs, lower workman's compensation costs, and fewer on- the- job accidents; a 75% reduction in inpatient substance abuse treatment costs after an EAP was implemented at Gillette; a McDonnell Douglas report, which estimated that its EAP saved the company $5.1 million due to fewer days missed from work, lower turnover, and fewer employee medical claims. The typical analysis of an EAP produces an ROI of between $3 and $10 dollars in return for every $1 dollar invested in the employee assistance program (EASNA, 2009).

In addition there is the question of legislative involvement in the promotion of pharmaceuticals as a solution for any kind of a medical, psychological, or psychiatric condition. Pharmaceuticals enjoy a unique position when it comes to the treatment of these conditions. At the present time there is no negotiation on the part of the federal government to reduce the cost of the pharmaceuticals from the brand name to the generics and even in the generics it is still very expensive.

So how did this happen? Congress to date has failed to allow for any negotiation on prices with Medicare. It's been estimated that the cost of pharmaceuticals in this country could be reduced by one third if not more if the federal government was allowed to negotiate the way private business can on its contracts. The position of the pharmaceuticals is that the reason you have to have the protection of the federal government is to protect the integrity of the medication itself. England and Canada, major English speaking countries, allow the government to negotiate prices on pharmaceuticals for their state run health plans.

The implication on the part of the pharmaceutical companies is that maybe the other countries don't care as much about the safety or efficacy of the medications as do the people in the United States. I will leave that to your discretion to determine if that's a valid argument.

Then, couple that with "how did this price arrangement occur?" Congress under the chairmanship of Representative Tauzin, a Congressman from Louisiana, was the chairman of the committee that held the hearings on pharmaceuticals being subject to negotiation. It was ruled at the time under his chairmanship that pharmaceutical prices were not to be negotiated by the federal government. Upon his leaving as Congressman, Representative Tauzin became the president of the Pharmaceutical Research and Manufacturers of America (PhRMA).

This is a perfect description of the BIG BOBBIE SHEELEY principle. The concept of this is that two major parties get together to the detriment of the public. This is an old folk expression that was used in the Honey Island swamp area where I grew up back in the 1920's and 30's. The Honey Island swamp originally was a pristine, cypress and hardwood land mass, separating the East and West Pearl River. The Great Southern Lumber Company and a major land owner, agreed to clear cut this treasure. The result was massive flooding to this whole area. It took 40 years for nature to restore itself. This example shows the consequences of the BIG BOBBIE SHEELEY principle and its significance remains today in the parallel to the modern day relationship with the federal government and the pharmaceutical industry. Let's just say that's it is not in the best interest of the public. Couple this dominance of non-negotiation with questionable TV advertising, the results are medical practice, insurance benefits, and legislation favoring the pharmaceuticals.

The mental health community has helped to create the illusion of the panacea of the magic bullet by virtue of the way they prescribe medications.

Historically, psychiatrists were therapists. However modern day practice of medicine precluded the psychiatrist from seeing the patient over a number of years because of the cost factor.

In Louisiana you couple that problem with the introduction of the medical psychologist which has created a whole new group of prescribing providers. Originally, as a lobbyist when this bill was introduced, I supported the psychologists because I felt it was an additional resource for the limited number of psychiatrists available at the time. The people that presented the program indicated that this would be a constraint on the number of medications and prescriptions written, time has proven this not to be true.

At a subsequent meeting I attended in Arizona, I met the author of this concept. He was a medical psychologist and had introduced this legislation and got it passed in Arizona. He came to Louisiana and I met him at the time the bill was introduced. In that meeting several years ago when he found out I was from Louisiana he told me if he had it to do over again he would never have introduced that bill because it added to the runaway costs of the pharmaceuticals with the advent of the medical psychologists.

Lest you think I am totally anti-pharmaceutical, let me cite you a couple of personal examples that have had a profound effect on my life. I have a sister, who at the age of 5 (1933) was diagnosed with acute pneumonia. I can remember the physician, Dr. Herbert Rothchild, coming out of the bedroom, this was in the days when physicians made house calls, and he told my mother the odds were that Jerrie would not make it through the night; except he may be able to get a new drug on the market called penicillin. Fortunately he was able to get the penicillin and started the medication on my sister that day. As a result she lived to be 74 years old. When I was in the Navy (1944) I contracted pneumonia and scarlet fever at the same time and was treated with the drug, penicillin. The doctors told me then it was the only thing that saved my life.

My issue is not with the physical medicine drugs but is the over prescription and mis-prescribed drugs for certain mental health conditions, i.e. depression, ADD, ADHD, bi-polar. For example, depression is currently treated with medication.

Studies going back as far as 1992 indicate that there is emerging documentation comparing effectiveness of talk therapy vs medication. These studies conducted by psychologists and neuroscience practitioners using non-evasive electromagnetic tests such as PET and fMRI looked at brain wave activity after talk therapy. The studies show that CBT or psychoanalytic therapy can be just as effective as medication. Such therapy can be more beneficial to the patient than the medication. This is where the real battle lies between therapy and pharmaceuticals. There are strong studies to indicate better outcome of cognitive behavioral therapy than medications. In view of the fact that there are serious challenges to the outcome of efficacy of medications to treat depression.

There is one other area that has had a profound effect on the use of medications. If you watch television you will see such programs as Dr. Oz, TVMD, or Ask a Doctor. All of these are social media types of medical practice. Many times people will take the comments that are made in a totally different way than the physician has intended it and use it to meet their own biases with respect to the use of the medication.

For example, I was working with a 16 year old diagnosed with ADD/ADHD (questionable diagnosis) and the question was whether he should be on Adderall. In my questioning of the mother of this teenager she reported that he had been off the Adderall for about 18 months and his grades had improved and his general behavior had improved. When the adolescent neurologist said to leave him off the Adderall, the mother said "oh no, you have to put him back on Adderall because that is what Dr. Oz says is needed if you are ADD/ADHD." The physician did put him back on Adderall. This is an example of the pressures that can be brought to bear on today's physicians.

So what other reasons are there for the pharmaceuticals to be so successful? If you watch the advertisements you will see the magic of the "sleight of hand." The whole time the description of the medication is being provided they usually start off with negative things but nothing serious, like you may bleed to death, you may commit suicide as a result of this, you may go blind, lose your hearing, and you may have an erection that lasts more than four hours and permanently ruin your sex life. That's the oral presentation of the medications with the cautions. If you watch the visual part of the advertisement you see a group of happy people, in wonderful settings, sea sides, anything that will distract you from the negative description of the pharmaceutical being described could cause. It's the old magician's way of being able to fool you into believing that his right hand is empty when he distracts you with his left hand and then all of a sudden the cards, scarf, or birds fly out of his right arm sleeve.

An example showing the impact of pharmaceuticals can be demonstrated with the large number of children and adolescents that were placed on Ritalin. Thirty years ago with the advent of the promotion and diagnosis of ADD/ADHD, Ritalin became the drug of choice for this condition. Even today there is a serious question about the diagnostic criteria used for this condition.

A personal example of this was an EAP case that I worked on involving a seven year old female in the second grade. The parents reported that she had become oppositional with respect to attending school. She refused to go to school. I met with the parents and Katie. Katie was a pretty, pig-tailed blonde, vivacious and animated, but also sad. When I asked her why she didn't want to go to school, she said "it makes me feel bad when the teacher calls me, Johnny, and Sarah up to the front of the class, and asks if we took our medicine". To which the teacher added "you know you are bad when you don't take the Ritalin". Katie replied "I'm not bad and I don't like what the teacher does".

I spent two hours with Katie doing what we call "walk therapy" –we did not conduct the interview in the office but rather in the park. This was done with her parents' permission and appropriate supervision. Clinically we find this setting less threatening to a child than an office setting designed for adults. Results–Katie was able to walk and talk with me for 2 hours, animated, but not hyper.

Her diagnosis had been based on the observation of the teacher, referred to a social worker, who then referred the child to a pediatrician. As it turned out none of these parties were trained in diagnosing ADD/ADHD. The end of the story is that Katie was reassigned to a different teacher and class and completed her elementary education without any further problems. I tracked this case until she graduated.

How many of your patients/clients are on medications? The odds are that many are on one or more. As therapists we can begin to change public attitude about behavioral health and treatment by asking our patients/ clients, "What medications are you taking? Follow that with "Is the medication working?" Many times you will find the answer is "I don't know", "I guess it is", or "I don't notice any difference". This is an opportunity to establish a relationship with the patients/clients prescribing physician. In your opinion and experience, is the medication actually improving or reducing the symptoms of the patient's condition?

The dilemma that we face as non-physicians was best explained in my story about Katie and the misuse of Ritalin. I am suggesting that you ask the patient if the medications are working. I am not suggesting that you attempt to advise your patients/clients about their medications. This is the responsibility of the prescribing physician.

The chapter on "Deep Capture" should raise serious questions to the American public and for you as a mental health practitioner and/or EAP counselor on your practice and your income.

CHAPTER 12

DEEP CAPTURE

This chapter addresses the signature question of "What the Hell is Behavioral Health?" It is the most controversial of all the data in this book. We have shown historically from the 1800's to 2005 what has been happening in the mental health and substance abuse field, i.e. the behavioral health field. We will document the various forces and how they are affecting not only public opinion, but also such entities as the FDA, medical practice by physicians, insurance companies, utilization review companies and EAP's. We will also demonstrate how businesses bought into the concept from an economic point of view and how that ultimately influences your practice and your income.

To show how this phenomenon is happening I will use the concept of "deep capture". First, I will define what the term "deep capture" means and why it's applicable in this case. "Deep Capture" was a term coined by Mark Mitchell, an investigative reporter with the Columbia School of Journalism, during his investigation of the securities market. Additionally, Patrick Byrne, founder and CEO of Overstock.com, picked up on this concept and wrote a blog explaining how this term is used to describe the capture and subsequent control of government or regulatory agencies by business or industry. The principle of Deep Capture is applicable to any kind of industry that has an impact on public opinion and is trying to influence how the public and governmental agencies will view these services and products.

If you are in the mental health or substance abuse field, you might ask what this term "deep capture" has to do with my practice, my income, and my patients. Let me explain why "deep capture" is so important. Ask yourself these questions: Is my practice any easier today than it was 5, 10, 15 years ago? Am I getting a better outcome with my clients/patients as a result of the innovative uses of drugs? If the pattern continues will my income increase or decrease? For those of us in the EAP field we will find that it has had a tremendous impact on the way we practice and deliver our services.

I consider myself to still be learning after 40 years of practice. I invite you to walk down the "deep capture" hall with me as we explore the different organizations that influence how we practice, how physicians prescribe, how medications are developed, how they are delivered to our clients, and how drugs are approved by the FDA.

I learned a long time ago that I need some sort of a check system to evaluate my thinking relative to what I am reading. If my thoughts and conclusions are different from what I am reading then I ask the question, can I trust the accuracy of what I am reading? I consider this to be an ongoing, learning process. Therefore, I ask you to look at the information presented and see if you come to similar conclusions about the state and direction of the mental health and substance abuse fields, i.e. behavioral health.

Let's start our journey of investigative reporting down the hall of "deep capture".

The first door we come to is marked PhRMA. PhRMA stands for Pharmaceutical Research and Manufacturers of America. Let's go inside and see what we can discover here.

There is a PhRMA webinar presentation showing the following information. "PhRMA's mission is to conduct effective advocacy for public policies that encourage discovery of important new medicines for patients by pharmaceutical and biotechnology research companies. To accomplish this mission, PhRMA is dedicated to achieving these goals in Washington, the states and the world:

- Broad patient access to safe and effective medicines through a free market, *without price controls*;
- Strong intellectual property incentives;
- And transparent, effective regulation and a free flow of information to patients.

PhRMA is devoted to advancing public policies in the U. S. and around the world that support innovative medical research, yield progress for patients today and provide hope for the treatments and cures of tomorrow."

PhRMA was formed in 1958 to represent America's biopharmaceutical research companies and "seek essential alignment between public policy and medical research to address patient needs."

Do you agree with my conclusion? PhRMA is a trade organization that is designed to influence public opinion, physicians practice, legislation, insurance benefits and promotion of its products without price controls. It is the funding device for many organizations that work to generate a favorable attitude toward the pharmaceutical industry.

As we continue down the hall, the next door we come to is labeled NAMI, which is one of the strongest advocacy groups in the mental health field. NAMI stands for National Alliance on Mental Illness.

As we enter this room there is a young volunteer describing NAMI's goals and activities. "This is a grass roots, family oriented, advocacy group that is designed to represent the best interests of the mentally handicapped or anyone with a mental health condition. NAMI relies on gifts and contributions to support our important work. The majority of our funding comes from individual donors and contributors and the remainder of our operations is financed by a variety of sources including corporate sponsorships, foundations, dues, grants, and partnerships."

The volunteer continues:

> "We educate families, individuals and educators to ensure they get the information and support they need. We advocate by shaping the national public policy landscape for people with mental illness and their families. We listen. There is a toll free helpline which allows us to respond personally to thousands of requests each year by providing free referral, information, and support.
>
> Anytime state or federal legislation affecting mental health (behavioral health) is being introduced we will have a strong turnout of the local NAMI chapter usually dressed in some sort of T-shirt identifying ourselves. We represent a strong vocal constituency that legislators will respond to."

Where does the principle of deep capture apply in this case? Where does the real funding for NAMI come from? Why PhRMA of course. Approximately 75% of all of NAMI's operating budget comes from money funded through PhRMA. If NAMI is representing the mental health field obviously they represent a strong force so PhRMA will fund their cause since it is in their best interest. This raises the question. What influence does PhRMA have within NAMI? Follow the money!

The next door that we encounter is labeled NIH (National Institute of Health). They are inviting us to come in and learn about the services and value of this organization. We learn that the NIH traces its roots to 1887 when a one room laboratory was created within the Marine Hospital Service. It was the predecessor agency to the U.S. Public Health Service. Their original mission was to promote the efficacy and improvement of patients' conditions. The NIH is an agency of the United States Department of Health and Human Services. It is the primary governmental agency responsible for biomedical and health-related research. They tell us that there are currently 27 different institutes within the framework of the NIH agency that do research in the health field. One of those 27 labs is the NIMH (National Institute of Mental Health). The NIMH is the largest research organization in the world specializing in mental illness. It was formed in 1949 by the federal government. Its mission is to "transform the understanding and treatment of mental illness through basic and clinical research, paving the way for prevention, recovery, and cure." NIMH is a $1.5 billion enterprise, supporting research on mental health through grants to investigators at institutions and organizations throughout the U. S. and through its own internal research effort. The NIMH represents the gold standard of practice used in treatment of different mental health conditions.

It is interesting to note, that almost every one of the studies performed under the auspices of NIMH involve the use of drugs. As evidence of the success of this program they cite a number of Nobel Prize winners in medicine that have been contributors to the NIMH. They also report on their website the successes of the people that have provided services for the NIMH such as in the polio vaccine. Following the introduction of the polio vaccine back in the 40's and 50's parents could finally go to bed at night without fear of waking up and finding their children being paralyzed.

So how does "deep capture" relate to the NIMH? First, the organization promoting its own self-interest produces a great deal of positive research. Next they invariably publicize the research in a favorable light. The research usually cites a number of studies that have been conducted by high profile academicians and high profile medical schools that have done research for the NIMH.

This generally raises a question of who funded the research for the individual studies. On the surface you will find that all the funding for NIMH is done by the federal government through Congressional approval. However, when you look at how these research papers are actually promoted, the money comes from the pharmaceutical companies. These are the very companies that are attempting to influence the decisions on the medications that are to be approved and prescribed.

The funding for these studies come from two separate sources, one from the federal government and one from the pharmaceutical industry itself. The funding process then raises two questions; is there a conflict of interest and can you trust the published research results? Remember all of this is focused toward one goal and that is to establish the "gold standard" for the treatment of any kind of mental illness or condition using a pharmaceutical.

If you follow the money, you will find that it all connects back to the researchers who are influenced to provide the right information so that the FDA will approve a particular drug. How much credibility can we actually give to the "gold standard rule" using pharmaceuticals as the panacea for these issues? Does this raise the question for how your clients/patients are being influenced to use medication instead of counseling?

As we continue our journey down the hall, the next door we encounter is labeled *Physicians' Desk Reference* or more commonly referred to as the *PDR*. We see that this book is published by the PDR Network, LLC in cooperation with participating manufacturers. What is the PDR and why is it important? The PDR is a commercially available compilation of manufacturers' prescribing information on prescription drugs. The PDR contains U.S. Food and Drug Administration (FDA) guidelines for the approved and non-approved use (off label) of each drug.

This is probably the most blatant example of "deep capture". Why? Who writes the description of the drug? The pharmaceutical company that manufactures the drug writes its own description of the benefits of the particular drug. For example, Hoffman-LaRoche who were the original manufacturers of Valium had about two to three columns on all the wonderful things Valium would do. It was presented as a panacea for everything from fallen arches to any type of mood disorder. At the very end of the description, but you have to read the whole thing, there is a warning which states "sudden abrupt withdrawal of the use of this drug may cause death." No serious consequences, right?

According to the FDA's guidelines, if a caveat or disclaimer has been issued for a particular drug it must be included in the description of the drug. However, there are any number of cases where that caveat has been totally ignored. The following information on "Johnson & Johnson" is documented through a series of articles taken from the Huffington Post, written by Steven Brill in 2016.

The "Johnson & Johnson" credo is "patients first, profits last". However, somewhere along the line, management changed this to emphasize profits to the detriment of people. While the investment analysts were hearing this wonderful story about the projected profits from their new drug "Risperdal", an Alabama teenage boy was awarded a $2.5 million settlement for damages when he developed 46DD breasts from using that drug.

The jury found that Johnson & Johnson had deliberately ignored the FDA warnings to not market or prescribe this drug to children, adolescents, or the elderly. It appears that management's decision to market Risperdal for off-label use of its product was in direct violation of FDA guidelines based solely on the strategy of "how much profit can we make to offset any legal actions?"

Johnson and Johnson was fined nearly $4.5 million in early 2009 for intentionally dispensing incorrect information about its Duragesic patches and anti-psychotic drug Risperdal. Eli Lilly agreed to pay $1.4 billion to settle allegations over illegal marketing practices relating to its schizophrenia and bipolar disorder treatment drugs. Pfizer agreed to pay $894 million to settle multiple lawsuits over alleged illegal marketing practices relating to its painkiller drugs, Celebrex and Bextra. GlaxoSmithKline paid $3 billion in fines for promoting its bestselling antidepressants for unapproved uses.

Whereas the Johnson & Johnson story is an example of greed at its worst, the next story is about arrogance at its best.

Before the Turing Pharmaceutical Company acquired the drug Daraprim, which is used to treat life threatening parasitic infections, the drug sold for $13.50 per pill. After Turing acquired Daraprim they increased the price of the drug to $750.00 per pill. This same drug sells for $2.00 in Europe. Remember the government is not allowed to negotiate its prices for Medicare/Medicaid pharmaceuticals.

There was a Congressional hearing on this particular price increase. Testimony indicated there was no change in the formula or research of this drug to justify this 50 fold increase. Howard Dorfman, legal counsel for Turing, warned CEO Martin Shkreli of this unjustified increase. Shkreli took Dorfman's advice by firing him. It is reported that Shkreli said to Dorfman "no one cares about price increases."

The next door we encounter is labeled *DSM-5 (Diagnostic Statistical Manual)*. As we enter, there is a representative from the American Psychiatric Association describing the history and use of the new DSM-5. This manual, first published in 1952, was called the DSM-1. It is now in its fifth revision. It was originally designed to describe the symptoms of the various psychological and psychiatric conditions which the mental health practitioner would then use to establish a diagnosis, severity of condition, and treatment plan.

In regards to physical medicine, the ICD-10 was designed to provide a method to describe a patient's condition and the basis of reimbursement for services. This program had over 6000 code articles that described the various medical conditions. Interestingly, there was not one code number that said the patient had no medical conditions.

With the new paradigm used under the DSM-5, the ICD-10 code is now used as the foundation to describe a patient's conditions and develop a diagnosis.

As an example of how convoluted and distorted a diagnosis can become we cite Premenstrual Dysphoric Disorder (PMDD). This a good example of the development of a non-existing DSM condition by the pharmaceutical companies which is designed to promote a new medication.

The inclusion of PMDD as a condition into the DSM came as a result of non-public group studies sponsored by pharmaceutical companies which were conducted by physicians, researchers, and representatives of the FDA. This group started in 1998 and subsequently recommended the condition be included in the DSM. PMDD was recognized as a disorder in 2013.

Within the medical community, there is ongoing severe criticism surrounding the study. The criticism is focused on the FDA's participation in meetings which were sponsored by the pharmaceutical companies. To treat the newly developed condition, the pharmaceutical industry brought pressure on physicians to prescribe Prozac for off label use. As a marketing ploy, they simply put a new dress on Prozac and called it Sarafem. An extensive television advertising campaign was then used to promote the new PMDD condition and Sarafem as a solution. This disorder has never been recognized in Europe because it doesn't stand up under independent study of symptoms and it doesn't demonstrate the efficacy of the antidepressants (Sarafem/Prozac) for the condition. This is a perfect example of pharmaceutical companies creating and promoting a new medication for a disease that doesn't even exist.

For an example of the dramatic change that occurred in the DSM-5 with the adoption of the medical model we can take a look at the description of grief.

As a therapist, you know there are a number of different forms of grief. Common forms are the loss of a loved one, divorce, loss of a job, etc. There are types of depression that are more medical in nature. However, the vast majority of grief issues reference the above examples. Under the DSM-5 medical model, grief is no longer a psychological problem. It is now a medical problem. So, if it is a medical problem, how do you treat medical problems? You medicate it. The new recommendation is that you treat depression with some sort of anti-depressant medication. As therapists you and I both know that if you shut down the grieving process, you have not solved the problem but simply delayed it which will likely create more problems in the future. So, how effective is the use of the medication? Long term, what is the best treatment of grief?

Does the new DSM-5 and the term "behavioral health" help us understand how to better diagnose and treat the patient? By changing definitions, we now use the term "substance use disorder" as a general classification rather than the old title of "alcoholism". The rationale for this change is that people who are struggling with alcoholism are less likely to use that term out of stigmatization. Is this true? Earlier we cited that numbers are growing worldwide for people seeking recovery through Alcoholics Anonymous. I think it would be difficult if not impossible for people who identify with AA to change from identifying themselves as "my name is Don and I'm an alcoholic" to "no identification and being a member of the substance use disorder club".

When we follow the money to see who owns and publishes the DSM, we find it's owned and published by the American Psychiatric Association (APA). The APA is an organization of psychiatrists formed to represent the political and economic interest of the psychiatric community.

What influence, if any, does PhRMA have on the American Psychiatric Association? How does PhRMA's influence affect the APA's official position?

How does it affect how the individual psychiatrist who prescribes drugs for treatment?

It is well documented that PhRMA has long recognized the need to have an influence at the most basic stage in the delivery of psychiatric services. How do you influence the most basic stage? You go to the medical schools where psychiatrists are trained. You pick the best teachers and you commission them to write favorable articles on a particular condition and drug. You can now cite a well-respected academic and a high profile psychiatrist as an authority on the condition and use of the drug.

It has been estimated that at least 70% to 80% of pharmaceutical reports have been ghost written by the so-called independent academic experts. Or as Fuller Torrey, executive director of the Stanley Foundation Research Programmes in Bethesda, Maryland put it "some of us believe that the present system is approaching a high class form of prostitution."

What documentation do we have as to what the actual influence of PhRMA is with the psychiatrists?

How can we determine the depth of influence PhRMA has within the American Psychiatric Association? If we follow the money we see, according to the APA, that 80% of its operating budget comes directly or indirectly from PhRMA.

Is there any professional organization or governmental regulatory agency that is not on PhRMA's assistance or influence list?

The last door we find down the "deep capture" hall reads SAMHSA. As we go through the door there is a representative giving the history of SAMHSA (Substance Abuse and Mental Health Services Administration). SAMHSA is a branch of the U.S. Department of Health and Human Services. It is charged with improving the quality and availability of prevention, treatment, and rehabilitative services in order to reduce illness, death, disability, and cost to society resulting from substance abuse and mental illnesses. SAMHSA evolved from a narcotics division in 1929 to the National Institute of Mental Health in 1973. In 1973 it became known as Alcohol, Drug Abuse, and Mental Health Administration (ADAMHA). In 1992 the new title of SAMHSA was created.

At the present time, it would appear that SAMHSA is the only governmental agency that is free of PhRMA's influence regarding the recommended use of drugs to treat mental health or substance abuse conditions. Free of

PhRMA's influence, SAMHSA has become the independent authority on the treatment of substance abuse and mental illness.

SAMHSA has recently issued a series of bulletins indicating there are questions related to the efficacy, outcome, and overuse of medications used to treat mental health and substance abuse problems. In response to SAMHSA questioning the use of drugs as therapy, the pharmaceutical industry and the American Psychiatric Association have launched a concerted attack against SAMHSA's position of using talk therapy instead of drugs.

The best analogy I can give you from a personal prospective is from World War II when we were in the Pacific and going to invade an island. The first action we took was to set up a barrage of artillery to soften up their positions. This was done with battle wagons standing 20 miles offshore and lobbing 2000 lb. shells into the enemy position. In my case I was flying a SB2C dive bomber and we were dropping 500 lb. bombs on these positions also. This analogy demonstrates what is happening in the attack on SAMHSA at the present time.

If we look at what the average psychiatrist does today we find they are no longer therapists. Their main function seems to be diagnosing, prescribing and managing medications based on the guidelines of PhRMA. Occasionally they will have a mental health practitioner on their staff, i.e. a social worker, deal with any talk therapy problems.

The purpose of "deep capture" is to gain control of the legislation and regulatory agencies that oversee your industry. If you want control you have to change attitudes and perceptions. One way to change attitudes and perception is to change the language. The choice of the term "behavioral health" is not random. I believe it was deliberately chosen to facilitate the shift to the medical/pharmaceutical model of treatment for the financial benefit of the pharmaceutical companies and to the detriment of society.

We no longer use the word alcoholism, instead we use the more general term of substance use disorder. We no longer treat grief as part of the human emotional and psychological experience; we now treat it as a behavioral dysfunction. By introducing the deliberately ambiguous term "behavioral health", the medical model can be used to prescribe drugs for every type of human behavior. If you are too happy we have a pill for that.

We now come back to the question "What the hell is behavioral health?" I maintain that "behavioral health" is a term that has no specific definition.

Having no definition allows each organization and discipline to define what it means and then promote their concept to their financial benefit.

Thought:

Who can you trust?

Who do you rely on for medical information?

Who do you and the public rely on or trust for information about drugs?

Who does the public rely on?

There are several things that I have trouble understanding or explaining. Is the universe expanding or contracting? How many galaxies are there? Are they dying or being born? I am not a scientist so I rely on astrophysicists and the Hubble telescope to explain these phenomenon.

What is the national debt? The treasury reported the national debt to be $19,232,950,841,710.63 or roughly $19 trillion. I don't know about you, but that doesn't fit my checkbook. We are told that the average debt per person in the United States (man, woman, and child), based on the 2013 census report, is $52,762.00. I can understand that number. Who is the authority on these numbers; is it the Treasury, the Budget Office, Congress or the Federal Reserve? Can I trust these sources to be accurate?

What is the cost of drugs and prescriptions? IMS Institute says spending on pharmaceuticals reached $424.8 billion in 2015. That amount is forecast to reach $640 billion in 2020 (I.M.S. Institute). It is estimated that spending on all prescription medicines will increase 22% by the year 2020 (I.M.S. Institute, 2016). An estimated $201 billion was spent in 2013 on mental disorders in the United States. This was more than any other medical condition. At least 26% of people in the United States are taking some sort of mental health drug. We know 25% of women are on anti-depressants and 11% of all Americans over the age of 12 are on anti-depressants. Anti-depressant medication is the third most common drug prescribed across all age groups. How many days, weeks, months, or years will the average person be medicated?

Who is the authority on prescriptions and can I believe them? The pharmaceutical association publishes data, Department of Health and Human Resources provides data, and companies like Express Scripts provide data. Can we believe all that they tell us?

This is where it gets personal.

Do you think the term "behavioral health" promotes the use of medication?

Have we unwittingly promoted the concept of behavioral health and the proliferation of medication? Have we allowed pharmaceuticals to establish a definition of the gold standard of treatment for mental health/substance abuse by the use of medications? How do you think "behavioral health" has affected your practice, the outcome of your patients and your income?

Chapter 13

Challenging the Status Quo

This is the last chapter to the book titled "What the Hell is Behavioral Health?" I will attempt to tie all the loose ends together and make some comments about what the future holds for our career as therapists based on what I see is happening in business, insurance, and legislation.

Man has always tried to predict the future. The best way to do that according to historians is to review the past. There have been many Greek and Roman quotations to admonish us to look to the past to see the future. And yet some of the real guides we use to look at the future are predictors like Nostradamus or the scripture as in the Apocalypse, or we can use the old fashioned fortune teller. How much more effective is the current predictability of the future than those espoused by the sometime accuracy or guesstimations of the fortune teller.

However, if we are to know what the future holds, the best way to predict that is to review the past. George Santayana summed it best by saying "those who do not learn history are doomed to repeat it". So at this point let's stop and review where we are, and what we have talked about, and what the predictions will be for the future based on the past. What is the future of the mental health and substance abuse counseling field and does the term "behavioral health" help in these predictions? The future can be either, very good or very bad, depending on the data that is reviewed, but I think it's important to view both the positive and negative before we attempt to make any conclusions on the future of our careers.

Over the last 20 years, the language of mental health and substance abuse has changed dramatically. As an example of that, one of the things I find interesting is the current use of the term "gold standard" to establish what is considered to be the best practices. That could range from pharmaceuticals to talk therapy of some kind. My question is "Who perfected the concept of the term "gold standard"? What were the standards used to establish the gold in the standard? To my knowledge I know of no one who has given us a real explanation for why we should automatically adopt the position that this is the best way to provide services. Again, my thesis this whole time has been to raise questions about what is happening. The expression "gold standard" is probably one of the better examples in the study of semantics because it connotes automatically the idea that something is good and valid and requires no further explanation.

When I reviewed the term "behavioral health", I asked clinicians and non-clinicians, what did that mean? The conclusion that I have drawn based on what the mental health field itself has said, is basically it means "what best serves my purposes today". Now those are my conclusions, drawn from those whom I have interviewed, especially if it has to do with the mental health practitioner. So, again, what is the value of the use of the term behavioral health? It only serves the purpose of the person or organization trying to establish their position in being the "gold standard" of treatment. The question is "do these two terms, "gold standard" and "behavioral health", truly improve the quality of care for our patients?"

The following is a brief review of some of the factors that influence the climate for the treatment of mental health and substance abuse in todays practice. Historically we have seen the use of mental health parity to describe something that was to be for the benefit of the mental health and substance abuse community. The concept was that it was unethical, if not illegal, to discriminate against one medical condition over another, i.e. you did not discriminate against medical conditions so why should you discriminate against mental health or substance abuse conditions. Somehow the concept of the differentiation of the brain separate from the rest of the body, makes no sense, when in fact the brain controls every part of the body.

Legislation has been drafted over the years to attempt to correct this discrimination, but in the acts themselves have perpetuated the discrimination against substance abuse because the bills were primarily for the benefit of mental health. The closest we have come in modern times to having a true mental health parity bill was in the ACA Obamacare plan. This said you could not discriminate against mental health and substance abuse and if the benefit was for 45 days then that's what you had to provide for both conditions. Even then there was discrimination in the machinations to control what the benefits would be regardless of how they were written.

One of the major areas that allowed the insurers to control the mental health and substance abuse benefits is the use of Utilization Review companies. Utilization Review companies came into existence in the late 1980's and began to flourish in the 1990's. These companies served a real purpose in that they attempted to establish a clinical standard that met the needs of the patient by diagnosis, site of service, severity of condition, and length of stay.

Do you view substance abuse as a separate and distinct diagnosis from any other condition? The old problem of the chicken or the egg, depression vs addiction, remains to be settled. However there are standards to establish which is primary. The Psychiatric Associations original decision tree on diagnosis states "unless you can establish the onset of the depression by 6 months prior to substance abuse issues, you cannot use this as a diagnosis". Yet you will see statistics that state 60% to 80% of patients suffer from a dual diagnosis condition. Our studies indicate the real number was closer to 25%.

However, all UR companies are not the same, many of them are used to hold down costs and deny services that are needed, i.e. if you have worked with a UR company that first asked "is the patient suicidal?", and if you said "no" then they said "they do not need to be in an inpatient treatment program". If this has been your experience with UR companies then you have been dealing with some of the less ethical groups. Many of the UR companies have served a good purpose to see that the patient received appropriate treatment, length of stay, and sites of service.

Case management is going to be used by the providers as a method of controlling costs from here on out, so you should understand how that works. Case management is the new term for an old service. Some insurers see the value of a follow-up service on appointments and medications to reduce readmissions for inpatient services and improve the quality of life for the patient. Case management can be a positive mutual support system for the therapists. Unfortunately in some instances it may also be an interference if not coordinated appropriately. However at the same time you want to make sure you have a working relationship with the UR companies which means you need to be prepared to document specifically why and how your patient is to be treated. If you provide the right information you will get the service you are requesting. If however you find you cannot get the services and it's not reasonable why your patient is being denied then you have the right and responsibility to inform your patient/client that they can appeal. The appeal process guarantees that there will be an independent review of the case and many times the original denial is overruled in favor of the patient.

One of the greatest barriers we have to mental health/substance abuse treatment is that of public attitude. Unfortunately many people still believe that mental health/substance abuse patient conditions are self- induced, and therefore do not meet or need any medical attention. We have a clinical and ethical responsibility to change this public opinion as much as we can through education and legislation. In addition, we as substance abuse practitioners should stop use of the term "disease concept" when describing substance abuse. Again what does this mean? It implies that somehow substance abuse is not a true disease, it is a reverse on semantics for what we are attempting to improve with insurance companies and public opinion. We never use the expression "disease concept" as in "cancer concept, or diabetes concept". Point made. It is either a disease or it is not.

Many physicians and mental health and substance abuse practitioners, myself included, decided to opt out of any insurance reimbursement plans. If you stop and think we have not made any great sacrifices. Most of the current insurance plans have huge deductibles and co-pays. The minimum deductibles are going to be around $2500.00 to $15,000.00. In most cases your client would never reach the deductible limit before the insurance company would start to pay and then you are only reimbursed after a substantial co-pay. Therefore you are in a position to give them the services they need without interference from an insurance company. If you were to review the monies being put into new treatment plans for mental health and substance abuse you will find there is a lot of new dollars being put into buying old treatment programs or establishing new treatment programs. The message here is: the investors believe that there is going to be a future in mental health/substance abuse in-patient and out-patient treatment programs. This is evidenced by the number of companies being formed or those that have been bought out.

There are many new telephonic systems that are being touted as the best use of time and money for the treatment of mental health/substance abuse, i.e. there is a battle going on within EAPA as to whether or not they should advocate or take an official position on telephonic or computer services in lieu of face to face interviewing. In line with that reasoning I would suggest that the federal government is in a position to evaluate the real value of face to face interviews. For example you cannot use telephonic or computer services if there is a question of a violation of the Drugs in the Workplace Act; i.e. positive drug test, that requires a face to face interview.

The greater the personal relationship exists between the counselor and the client, the more likely your career is going to be advanced and you will get a better outcome for your patient.

Add to this mix the current attempt at revision to the ACA Obama Health Care Plan that is currently transpiring in Congress. One of the most interesting and unfortunate things happening is described by the committee hearings in which it was reported that one of the committees in the House suggested that they bring in an actuary to determine the true costs of the health plan revisions rather than an estimate based on their opinions. This was brought up as a result of the discussions about the fact that you could not have any pre-existing conditions that would deny a patients right to coverage. It would seem to me that this would have been an earlier discussion about costs, and that established what the premiums would be, based on what the claims are. These are the kinds of issues and attitudes that make you stop and think about what the plan will look like coming out of Congress?

One of the major concerns along with the coverage for un-insurable's is making mental health/substance abuse an optional benefit. If this happens it will be a continuation of the discrimination against mental health and substance abuse.

One of the problems currently facing us is the use of medications in lieu of counseling. In my own case I ask every patient what medications are you on, why are you on it, and how is it working? It's amazing that I get responses to the last question like "it's working, I guess it's working, I don't know if it's working". Here is an opportunity for you to have a conversation with the treating physician. This is also an opportunity for you to show that you truly have a service to provide by sharing important information.

Regardless of why they come in, I always administer the PHQ-9 depression scale, which gives me an accurate description of where the patient is clinically and that information can be helpful to the physician about whether to continue, reduce, or eliminate the medication.

If there is a change in the atmosphere, physicians begin asking questions about mental health and substance abuse and are more likely to listen if we give them a clinical description of what the patient is and show them we can be joint partners in providing the best services for our mutual patient.

The other area we need to be more involved in is the education of the business community and insurance underwriters. If we are to be successful we have to demonstrate the efficacy of what we do and what we do produces a better outcome. Not many of the pharmaceuticals that are promoted will give you outcome studies on the patients using their medications. If you do not ask questions about the improvement or current status from the time your patient came to see you, with an ongoing questionnaire, then you are missing the boat. You need to review that the patient's treatment plan is on track.

One of the major areas to promote our position is through the education of the health insurance agents. The agents are interested in providing the best information for their clients so that they can maintain that relationship. We work with a select group of agents to make sure they know we are in a position to give them information relative to the best use of mental health and substance abuse benefits of their plans. In line with the broker services, one of the questions employers are interested in is "what return on investment documentation is there to demonstrate that I should buy or expand my mental health and substance abuse benefits?"

There are many studies that are available, some we have done on our own, some we have reviewed with national organizations, to document return on investment of the recommendations that we make.

In summary, what is the predictable future for the mental health and substance abuse field? If we continue to allow the pharmaceuticals and non- mental health practitioners to dictate how mental health services are going to be provided, you are fighting a losing battle. However, based on suggestions made here, we feel that we are in a strong position to enhance the proof of the value of mental health and substance abuse benefits. We should take charge of the term "behavioral health" and give it a specific definition as to what it deserves. It has to do with the mental faculties, functionality of our clients, as well as their use or misuse of substance abuses and how that is affecting their lives and their families. If we take charge of these areas of responsibility, we should be in a position to change the definition of behavioral health to one more specific to our practice and our client's diagnosis. The correct use of the diagnosis of mental, nervous, or substance abuse disease will give us a better description of the patient's needs. Finally it gives us a true picture of the fallacy of the use of the term "behavioral health."

Ethics- so what is your license? Is it academic training in mental health or substance abuse? Do you have the academic and experiential service necessary to practice in the addiction field? Most mental health practitioners have never been trained in substance abuse. If you practice in the mental health field, what is your attitude toward dual diagnosis? Does the lack of specific training, academic and experience in substance abuse, create an ethical problem in providing services for the substance abuse client/patient?

The term "behavioral health" should challenge the prevailing view that the mind is separate from the other organs of the body. Until we understand and accept that the brain controls all parts of the body and cannot be excluded for medical purposes. (It is not when the heart stops beating when the patient has died, it is when the brain wave activity cease that the patient is pronounced medically dead.) The early Greeks and native Shamans understood the mind-body concept which they described as spirits.

Throughout this book I have asked the question "What the Hell is Behavioral Health?" In conclusion, I offer the following definition in answer to that question. It is an interdisciplinary approach to prevent, educate, diagnose and treat illness of the mind, body, and spirit.

Book References

Chapter 1 – The Telephone Call
   1-Interview with Nancy Gwaltney, January 30, 2015

Chapter 2 – My Life Experiences

Chapter 3- Interventions: Mine and Others
   1-Johnson, Vernon, "I'll Quit Tomorrow", Harper One, 1980.

Chapter 4 – History of Alcohol
   1-Whiskey Speech, The Clarion Ledger, February 24, 1996, Jackson
      Mississippi.
   2-History of Wine, https://en.wikipedia.org/wiki/History_of_wine
   3-History of Beer, https://en.wikipedia.org/wiki/History_of_beer
   4-The History of Amber Nectar, http://www.history-of-beer.com/
   5-History of Alcoholic Beverages, http://en.wikipedia.org/wiki/His-
      tory_of_alcoholic_beverages
   6-Alcohol: A Short History, http://www.drugfreeworld.org/drugfacts/al-
      cohol/a-short-history.html
   7-Ditty- http://www.newyorkcarver.com/wine.htm
   8-Samoset- https://en.wikipedia.org/wiki/samoset
   9-Have You Got Any Beer, the Paracast Community
      Forums,http://www.theparacast.com/forum/threads/history-les-

son—have-you-got-any-beer.3006/

10-Fleet, Anna, 10 Ways Drinking Beer Can Help Save Your Life, Active Beat,http://www.activebeat.co/yourhealth

11-Volstead Act – http://www.nolo.com/legal-encyclopedia/content/prohibition-act.html

12-Black Death- https://en.wikipedia.org/wiki/Black Death

13-History of Alcohol Distillation -http://www.copper-alembic.com/ns/cms/php?id_cms=26

14-Wine In The Ancient World-http://churchhistory101.com/wine-alcohol-bible.php

15-History and Taxonomy of Distilled Spirits, June 19, 2002,http://www.alexreisner.com/misc/distilledspirits

16-The Gin Epidemic – http://alcalc.oxfordjournals.org/content/36/5/401

17-Gin History, Development and Origin, http://www.ginvodka.org/history/ginhistory.asp

18-The Best Invention Since the Wheel – https://www.arenaflowers.com/wine_club_online?history_of_wine

19-A Brief History of Wine, The New York Times, November5, 2007, http://www.nytimes.com2007/11/05/timestopics/topics-winehistory.html?_r

20-Cheers to the Magna Carta, http://magnacarta800th.com/events/beer-day-britain/

21-Amendments – https://alcoholpolicy.niaaa.nih.gov/About_Alcohol_Policy.html

22-Spiess, DJ, Thanksgiving, Pilgrims, and Beer Myths, Fermenterium, http://www.fermenterium.com/random-news/thanksgiving-pilgrims-and-beer-myths/

23-King James Version -1 Corinthians 6:10

24-Carry Nation Smashed Bar, http://www.history.com/this -day-in history/carry-nation-smashes-bar

25-Volstead Act, Encyclopedia Britannica

26- Alcohol by Volume, https://en.wikipedia.org/wiki/Alcohol_by_volume

27- Franciscus Sylvius, https://en.wikipedia.org/wiki/Franciscus_Sylvius

28- 11 Perfectly Good Reasons to Drink More Gin, https://thoughtcatalog.com/natalie-morin/2014/08/11-perfectly-good-reasons-to-drink-more-gin

29- Guisepi, Robert, The History of Ancient Sumeria, 1980 and 2003, http://history-world/sumeria.htm

Chapter 5 – Grapers, Inebriates, Alcoholics, and Substance Abusers

1-White, William, Slaying The Dragon, Chesnut Health Systems, 2014

2- National Institute on Drug Abuse, March 2011, https://www.drugabuse.gov/publications/drugfacts/treatment-statistics

3- Williams, Trish, Losing Tom, Alcoholism –A Disease, 7/29/16, http://www.losingtom.org/alcoholism/disease.html

4- Screedler, Update on the Jellinek Curve, 3/18/12,http://discoveringalcoholic.com/update-on-the-jellinek-curve/

5-Magnus Huss, http://todayinsci.com/H/Huss_Magnus/HussMagnusQuotations.htm

6- Hersey, Brook, The Controlled Drinking Debates: A Review of Four Decades of Acrimony, April 2001.

7- Peele, Stanton, Through a Glass Darkly, Psychology Today, April 1983.

8- Brief History of the Controlled Drinking Controversy, Medscape,http://www.medscape.com/viewarticle/473554_2.

9-Sobell, Linda and Mark, Individualized Behavior Therapy for Alcoholics, June 2006, http://www.sciencedirect.com/science/article/pii/S0005789473800747

10- Boffey, Phillip, Showdown Nears in Feud Over Alcohol Studies, The New York Times, November 2, 1982.

11- Westermeyer, Robert, Harm Reduction and Moderation, http://www.addictioninfo.org/articles/233/1/Harm-Reduction-and-Moderation/Page1.html.

12- Keeley Institute, https://en.wikipedia.org/wiki/Keeley_Institute

13- Mandros, Athena, A New Era In Addictions: Medication Assisted Treatment, Open Minds, April 28, 2016.

Chapter 6 – Evolution of the EAP

1-White, William, The Evolution of Employee Assistance: A Brief History and Trend Analysis

2- The Rockefeller Dinner, http://www.barefootsworld.net/aarockdinner.html

3- Conversation with Bob Jones, July 22, 2015

4- Conversation with Greg DeLapp, July 20, 2015

5- Mansfield, Stephen, The Search for God and Guinness: A Biography of the Beer that Changed the World. July 8, 2014

6- Harold Hughes: Clean and Sober Recovery Hero Addiction Alcoholic,
http://www.cleanandsobernotdead.com/recoveryhero/hughes.html.

Chapter 7 – Not My Job

Chapter 8 – Legislation

1-State Mental Illness Parity Laws, NAMI,
http://lobby.la.psu.edu/006_coverage_parity/organizational_statements/nami/nami_state.htm

2-The Wellstone-Domenici Mental Health Parity Act of 2008: Questions and answers for psychologists, http://www.apapracticecentral.org/news/2008/wellstone-domenici.aspx

3-Levin, Bruce, The Louis de la Parte Florida Mental Health Institute, Mental Health Parity: National State Perspectives 1998, University of South Florida, Tampa, Florida

4-Mental Health Parity Laws by State, Insure.com,May 5, 2010,
http://www.insure.com/health-insurance/mental-laws-by-state.html

5-Szalavitz, Maia, When the Cure Is Not Worth the Cost, New York Times, April 11, 2007, http://www.nytimes.com/2007/04/11/opinion/11szalavitz.html?ei=5070

6-Enos, Gary, Survey: Public Strongly Supports Less Criminalization of Addiction, Addiction professional, January 27, 2016

7-CMS Final Medicaid Parity Rule Released, Open Minds, April 3, 2016, https://www.openminds.com/market-intelligence/news/cms-releases-final-medicaid-rule-mental-health-addiction-treatment-parity.htm/

8-Millhollon, Michelle, Legislature Oks 99-Year Sentence for Heroin

Dealers,
http://www.theadvocate.com/baton_rouge/news/politics/legislature/article

9-Legiscan, https://legiscan.com/LA/bill/SB271/2016

10-Opioid Epidemic Plagues Workers Comp, Insurance Journal, May 17, 2013,
http://www.insurancejournal.com/news/national/2013/05/17/292522
8.htm

11-Overview of US Medical Marijuana Law, http://www.medicalmarijuanainc.com/overview-of-u-s-medical-marijuana-law.

12 – Social Norms are Changing Regarding the Use of Marijuana, Introventions, November 14, 2016,

13- Senators Domenici and Wellstone Introduce Mental Health Equitable Treatment Act of 1999, NAMI,
http://lobby.la.psu.edu/006_Coverage_Parity/Organizational_Statements.

14- History of Unites States Drug Prohibition,
https://en.wikipedia.org/wiki/History_of_United_States_drug_prohibition.

15- Futch, David, How Marijuana Legalization Could Affect Employers Drug Testing Policies, L.A. Weekly, July 18, 2016.

Chapter 9 –Feeding The Dragon

1-How Life Expectancy Has Varied Over The Past 100 Years, Get Holistic Health, October 15, 2012,
http://www.getholistichealth.com/8129/how-life-expectancy-has-varied-over-the-past-100-years

2-How Has Life Expectancy Changed Over Time? September 9, 2015,
http://visual.ons.gov.uk/how-has-life-expectancy-changed-over-time/

3- Heneghan, Carolyn, Healthcare Journal of Baton Rouge, September/October 2016, Price Is Right

4-A History of Blue Cross and Blue Shield,
http://www.bcbs.com/blog/health-insurance.html

5-How Much Does an Appendectomy Costs?
http://health.costhelper.com/appendicitis.html

6-Cost of an Appendectomy? http://www.cbsnews.com/news/cost-of-an-appendectomy-reddit-user-posts-55000-bill/

7-Waguespack, Stephen, Presidents View: Take the Time to Do it Right, LABI Communications, January 31, 2017.

8-Four Mega Trends Driving Sustainability In the Mental Health Market, Open Minds, July 19, 2017

9-Reinhardt, Uwe, New York Times, September 25, 2009, How Much Money Do Insurance Companies Make? A Primer,http://economix.blogs.nytimes.com/2009/09/25/how-much-money-do-insurance-companies-make.

10- Health Care in the Unites States, https://en.wikipedia.org/wiki/Health_care_in_the_United_States

11-The History of Health Insurance in the United States, http://www.neurosurgical.com/medical_history_and_ethics/history/history_of_health_insurance

12-About Willow Bark Tea, http://www.gardenguides.com/93937-willow-bark-tea.html

13-Marigold, http://www.home-remedies-for-you.com/herbs/marigold.html

14- A Short History of Medical Insurance

15- The Cost of Having a Baby in the United States, Medscape, October 3, 2016.

16- CMS.gov, August 2014, https://www.cms.gov/Research-Statistics-Data-and-Systems/Statistics-Trends-and-Reports

17-IMS Institute for Healthcare Informatics, 2015.

18- Berkrot, Bill, U.S. Prescription Drug Spending to Hit $400 Billion a Year by 2020, AHIP Solutions Smartbrief, April 15, 2016.

19- Harding, Fran, Strategic Initiative #1, A Plan For SAMHSA's Role and Actions http://www.cdc.gov/workplacehealthpromotion/evaluation/topics/depression

20-Medicine Use and Spending Shifts, IMS Health, National Sales Perspectives, December 2014; National Prescription Audit, January, 2015.

21-Bindley, Katherine, Women and Prescription Drugs, November 16, 2011, http://www.huffingtonpost.com/2011/11/16/women-and-presciption-drug-use_n_

22- Antidepressant Rankings, http://www.sfgate.com/health/article/Antidepressants - nation-s-top-prescription-4034392

23-Medicines Use and Spending in the US, IMS Institute for Healthcare Informatics, April 2016.

24-The Economic Burden of Mental Illness, Florida Council for Community Mental Health, www.fccmh.org.

25-Klachefsky, Michael, Hidden Costs, Productivity, Losses of Mental Health Diagnosis, Benefits Magazine, February 2013.

26- Depression and Lost Productivity, University of Michigan Depression Center, 2016, http://www.depressioncenter.org/work/information-for-employers/lost-productivity.

27- National Institute on Drug Abuse, March 2011, https://www.drugabuse.gov/publications/drugfacts/treatment-statistics

28- Health Insurance in the United States, https://en.wikipedia.org/wiki/Health_insurance_in_the_united_states

Chapter 10 – Factors Influencing Diagnosis/Reimbursement

1-What is Dual Diagnosis, Addiction Center, https://www.addiction-center.com/addiction/dual-diagnosis/

Chapter 11 – Pharmaceuticals

1-Schwartz, Casey, Generation Adderall, The New York Times Magazine, October 12, 2016, http://nytimes.com/2016/10/16/magazine/generation-adderall-addiction.html?

2-Whitaker, Robert, Anatomy of An Epidemic, Crown Publishers, New York, 2010.

3- Sears Roebuck Catalog, 1897, pg. 41.

4- The Coleman Institute, January, 2016, Did the Crackdown on Doctors Writing So Many Prescriptions Cause the Dramatic Increase in Heroin Use?

5-Who is the Father of Pharmacy?, https://www.quora.com/Who-is-the-father-of-pharmacy

6-Smith, Brendan, Inappropriate Prescribing, American Psychological Association, June 2012

7-Insel, Thomas, Antidepressants: A Complicated Picture, NIMH, December 6, 2011, http://www.nimh.nih.gov/about/director/2011/an-tidepressants

8- Ehrlich Finds Cure for Syphilis, LPB, http://pbs.org/wgbh/aso/data-bank/entries/dm09sy.html.

9 – Harding, Fran, Strategic Initiative #1, SAMHSA's Roles and Actions

10- Billy Tauzin, http://epicroadtrips.us/2003/summer/nola/nola_offsite

11 – Hoyt, M.F. (2017). Brief Therapy and Beyond: Stories, Language, Love, Hope, and Time, Routledge Publishing, New York: Routledge.

12- Cummings, N.A. Psychology's Soothsayer, 2013.

13- Cummings, N.A. (2000,2002) The Collected Papers of Nicholas A. Cummings (Vols. 1 and 2, ed. By J.L. Thomas & J.L. Cummings). Phoenix, AZ: Zeig, Tucker, Theisen.

14- Cummings, N. A., & O'Donohue, W.T. (Eds., 2011). Understanding the Behavioral Healthcare Crisis: The Promise of Integrated Care and Diagnostic Reform. New York: Routledge.

15- Hoyt, M.F. (1995). Brief Therapy and Managed Care. San Francisco: Jossey-Bass.

16- Hoyt, M.F. (2000). Some Stories Are Better than Others: Doing What Works in Brief Therapy and Managed Care. New York: Brunner/Mazel.(now Routledge)

17- EAP Effectiveness and ROI, EASNA Research Notes, Volume 1, Number 3, October 2009.

18- EAPs Save Companies Money, EA Industry Spotlight, March 2016.

19- Overprescribing Drugs to Treat Mental Health Problems. Psychology Today, January, 2014.

Chapter 12 – Deep Capture

1-Pollack, Andrew, The New York Times, February 4, 2016, Drug Firms Expected to Defend Huge Price Increases in House Testimony

2-Fauber, John, Medpage Today, November 16, 2016, Lowering the Bar: How PMDD Went from an Idea to a Diagnosis

3-Annual Causes of Death in the United States, http://www.drugwar-facts.org/chapter/causes_of_death

4-Overdose Death Rates, National Institute on Drug Abuse, January

2017, https://www.drugabuse.gov/related-topics/trends-statistics/overdose-death-rates

5- Fox, Maggie, Heroin Deaths Quadruple Across U.S., July 7, 2015, http://www.nbcnews.com/pages/print

6-Byrne, Patrick and Mitchell, Mark, The Story of Deep Capture, 2014

7-About PhRMA, http://www.phrma.org/about

8- About NIMH, http:/www.nimh.nih.gov/about/index.shtml

9- About NAMI, http:/www.nami.org/About-NAMI

10- National Institute of Mental Health, https://en.wikipedia.org/wiki/National_Institute_of_Mental_ Health

11- National Institute of Mental Health, http://www.nih.gov/about-nih/what-we-do/nih-almanac/

12- About the Physicians' Desk Reference

13- Substance Abuse and Mental Health Services Administration, https://en.wikipedia.org/wiki/Substance_Abuse_and_Mental_Health_Services_Administration

14_ Using DSM-5 in the Transition to ICD-10, http://www.dsm5.org/Pages/Default.aspx

15- Brill, Steven, Backstage at Johnson & Johnson, Huffington Post, http://highline.huffingtonpost.commiracleindustry/americas-most-admired-lawbreaker/chapter -1.html

16- Boseley, Sarah. Scandal of Scientists Who Take Money for Papers Ghostwritten by Drug Companies, The Guardian, February 2002.

17- Whitaker, Robert. Anatomy of an Epidemic, Crown Publishers, New York, 2010, pg. 278.

18- Grohol, John, NAMI: Nearly 75 Percent of Donations from Pharma, World of Psychology.

19- List of Pharmaceutical Settlements, https://en.wikipedia.org/wiki/List_of_largest_pharmaceutical_settlements.

20- Perrone, Matthew, Lawmakers Challenge Turing Executives on Drug Price Hikes, The Washington Post, https://www.washington-post.com/business/lawyer-turing-execs-warned-shkreli-against.

21- Competitor to Offer $1 Pill After Turing Price Hike Outrage, NBC News, October 22, 2015.

22- Drug Firms Expected to Defend Huge Price Increases in House

Testimony, February 4, 2016,
https://www.pharmacist.com/node/971740.

23- Bakalar, Nicholas, Drug Company Lunches Have Big Payoffs, The New York Times, June 20, 2016.

24- Roethel, Kathryn, Antidepressants – Nations Top Prescription, SF-GATE.

25- Outlook to 2020, Medicine Use and Spending in the US, IMS Institute for Healthcare Informatics

26- Hroncich, Caroline, IMS Institute Examines Medicine Use and Spending in 2015, http://www.pharmtech.com/ims-institute-report-examines-medicines.

27- Largest Share of Health Spending is on Mental Disorders, Health-Leaders media News, June 14, 2016.

Chapter 13 – Challenging The Status Quo

1- Behavioral Health, mediLexicon, http://www.medilexicon.com/dictionary/39449

2- Quote, George Santayana, http://bigthink.com/the-proverbial-skeptic/those-who-do-not...

3- Quotes, http://www.goodreads.com/quotes/tag/doomed-to-repeat-it

4- Making A Diagnosis, American Family Physician, October 15, 1998, http://www.aafp.org/afp/1998/1015/afp19981015p1347-fl.gif

www.ingramcontent.com/pod-product-compliance
Lightning Source LLC
Chambersburg PA
CBHW070657290526
45790CB00001B/363